Sister Stories

Breaking the Silence of Menopause.

Angela Reeves

DEDICATION

This book is dedicated to my soul sister and bestie for life,
Kim Wright, the person who taught me that it isn't what you have in your
life that matters, it's who you have in your life.
♥

CONTENTS

ACKNOWLEDGMENTS

I gratefully acknowledge the bravery of every person who has shared their story publicly for the benefit of others, creating this volume of valuable truths. If we only help one other woman by sharing our truth, it will be worth the effort. Much love and respect to you all.

PART 1
THE MAKING OF SISTER STORIES

I don't remember anyone ever explaining menopause to me before it happened. Not ever. When it started for me I had maybe heard some older ladies complaining of hot flashes, but it never really occurred to me that this was in any way relevant to me, having just turned 40. I had a vague notion that this was some relatively uncommon thing that "older" ladies liked to bitch about, but I never really considered that perhaps this was something that I needed to know about, not at the time anyway.

When I realized with a shock just after 40 that I WAS menopausal, I kept having a recurring thought, very clear & direct - glowing like neon in front of my eyes every time I had a hot flash - why the hell didn't somebody tell me this was coming?

We are in an age of medical information enlightenment and extreme ease of sharing of information. Somebody forgot to tell menopause that.

We teach all our youngsters about the changes that are coming with adolescence & sexuality, we coach our young women every step of the way through their periods & PMS.   Mothers to be are as uber educated as their doctors and midwives about the before, during and after both physically and mentally with pregnancy. Postpartum isn't a dirty word any more, neither is period - men generally no longer run away vomiting at the thought of it, and all those things have become very acceptable aspects to life in polite society.

So what the F*** could be the possible reason we don't properly prepare & inform 50% of our population about what is the largest & longest physical transition of their lives, and what has the longest list of potentially life altering symptoms of any time in the female lifespan. Forget periods & PMS, move aside childbirth - menopause trumps it all - and best of all as a special bonus - it can last a decade or more. (I have a personal theory that a huge percentage of midlife divorce is a direct result of menopause and our inability to cope with it, talk about it and understand it - as women, and often as couples.)

So with that question flashing neon every day - why the hell didn't somebody tell me this was coming? I began reaching out and talking with other women, trying to learn everything I could about the range of experiences of as many women as possible. Turns out, nobody really told any of them it was coming either, and many of them were experiencing real angst & confusion similar to mine. Many admitted to feelings of isolation or shame when it came to discussing the topic at all.   **It was that recurring fact that drove me to write this book.** My hope is to give even one woman the sense that what she is feeling is not unique to her alone, that she is normal and ok and there is nothing wrong, maybe it's not you, maybe it's menopause and it's high time we shared our truths.

How it was for me:

I think on the general spectrum of menstrual matters, I was kind of medium.   4 - 5 day periods, heavy the first 2 days, lighter the rest.   Medium cramps, maybe a bit more than medium PMS.   Nothing really out of the ordinary or spectacular to report about my experience to that point. Physically I'm also pretty much medium.   Neither, fat or skinny, just kind of in between, moderately fit, moderately active, moderate to high stress levels personally & professionally.

I probably was what they call "peri" menopausal from about 35, not that it affected me much.   My periods just kind of dwindled away, becoming more and more irregular.   I'm not sure how long it was actually, but the first time I noticed a long pause, I did the count back and realized I hadn't had a period for 9 months, I was 39.   Then I got a doozie that lasted a week and a half, reminding me that my inner works were still "working". After that I think there was about 11 months of nothing, and then about a year of fairly regular periods before a full year of nothing.   Anyone who has checked in with a doctor will likely be told the same thing I was, that until you go a full calendar year without one, they don't really bother to do the blood work to confirm with hormone levels. I was in a new relationship just after 40, in a sexual "second spring" as I fondly recall it, and I remember a few fretful months when the periods didn't come (even though my partner is one of the tiny % of men who do the after testing to confirm their vasectomy) of perhaps a miracle pregnancy? Of course none of that was in the cards, we were well past it, and didn't know it. A flat line blood hormone test confirmed I was indeed fully menopausal. The only babies coming my way would be future grandbabies. I guess I was fine with that, but I did feel a little part of me curl up and die feeling I was past date, and my eggs were expired.

Don't get me wrong - I LOVED not having a period anymore, so much so, that even though my symptoms were bad for a long time, I pushed that aside and embraced the gratitude for no more cramps or leaks or any of that period crap. How lovely. But the insomnia, anxiety and the constant profuse unexpected all over my body sweats weren't such a good trade, as I soon found out.

It was pretty much all at once that I started noticing the differences in my body without hormones. I went from being kind of "medium" in my feminine matters to definitely not medium.   Having ALWAYS been a very sound sleeper, I began to experience insomnia for the first time in my life, and I learned to get by on perhaps 3 or 4 hours of cumulative unconsciousness in a night. Much like having a newborn in the house, wandering around in a vague fog of exhaustion for months. Hot flashes followed with intensity shortly thereafter, exacerbating the insomnia. They came in a fury so intense and so frequent I couldn't bear it any longer, and after about 6 months of burning in my own personal hell, I decided to talk to my doctor about seeking refuge in HRT. (Any moisture in the nether regions also dried up making sex uncomfortable at best on the rare occasions I offered any up). Over the last 10 years, I did 2 separate rounds of HRT, each for about 2 years, and going off each time because of diminishing efficacy (I was iffy about hormones in general and refused to increase my dosage.

Over the years I've tried a lot of different herbals, with varying degrees of success, as well as changes to diet (bye bye red wine, see ya later red meat!), acupuncture, had cardiac testing for the heart palpitations (where the technician said - "oh, your heart rate doesn't change during a hot flash, that's just in your head".)   Nothing I've tried has been the golden ticket, but certain things have helped me, most notably melatonin & magnesium for sleep.

For years I felt angry and frustrated ALL the time.   Not depressed, nor anxious, but really, really angry, and not really sure why.   I didn't tell anyone what was happening as I was in such sad shape from the insomnia, I didn't even really register what was happening to the point I could express it properly.   I think there's still a huge stigma towards the aging woman and we are somehow rendered less by our loss of fertility in the eyes of "society".   So for these and whatever other reasons I just stayed quiet and didn't share my strange internal goings on with anyone.

There was a vague notion in me that I wasn't depressed or anxious, but this feeling was altogether as powerful and intense, but it felt very different than any anxiety or depression I had felt before.   I was just so very ANGRY and in my more lucid moments I was pretty convinced I was losing my marbles.

I am currently in my twelfth year of contending with insomnia & never ending hot flashes and night sweats.   Thankfully, the anxiety has lessened and I no longer wake up feeling panicked in the middle of the night.   I still have heart palpitations, usually once an evening, but I long ago became accustomed to all of it.   I hope I am almost at the end of the tough part of this road!!

How this book physically came to be:

The only good part of profusely sweating at random moments is that it is a great icebreaker to a conversation about menopause!!   I owned a gift and flower shop for several years and had occasion to speak with hundreds of women from every walk of life so I made good use of the opportunity.   If I could turn sweat dripping off my temples and running in lines down my ribs into an intro to a learning opportunity or a personal connection, at least I could get something out of it besides embarrassment!!

Turns out, not very many women that I encountered know very much more than I did about menopause, and many were initially a bit put off by any inquiries I gently put forward about their experience.   Luckily, I'm blessed with good listening skills, and people tend to open up to me easily & I was delighted and enthralled to hear every funny story or horrible detail each women had to share.   I talked to a lot of women my age and older, and later I began to ask younger women what they knew about what was coming.   They generally didn't know squat either.

One of the key moments for me in this process was an amazing conversation I had with a relative stranger in my shop one afternoon.   She had spent a nice long while browsing on a quiet afternoon in the shop, we had exchanged some chit chat & she had come up to the counter & I was packaging her selections & wrapping her flowers.   As it went in those days, I got hit with maybe the 10th hot flash of that hour, and she noticed sweat running down my forehead and asked me if I was ok.   I laughed it off with my usual line "the eternal flame of menopause is just burning within me". I think she would have been about late 50's in age, and she was surprised that someone as "young" as I was would even know about it, let alone have it.   We exchanged some stories and I asked her, "What would you say has been the worst part about menopause for you?"   She took a cautious look over each shoulder to ensure we were alone and she wouldn't be overheard. I'll never forget what she said.   "Do you really want to know?" asked the very proper looking schoolteacher "Well, I'll tell you what the worst thing is for me, it's the FUCKING RAGE."   I was pretty surprised, she didn't look the type to me to have rage, much less admit it- but she voiced exactly what I felt but had never defined so well in myself. Turns out, she wasn't unique within her circle at the school, and she shared the running joke from her principal which was that the 5 or 6 female teachers "of a certain age" should put out some kind of red flag by their classroom doors as some kind of hazard warning system.

That was the moment I realized that the powerful feelings of anger (actually, the FUCKING RAGE!!)I had been experiencing were actually a part of menopause.   That was a game changer.   I became intensely interested in learning the stories of as many women as possible to expand my information base about exactly what menopause is, and the many different ways it can feel.   I met so many relatively young women (who were likely perimenopausal and didn't know it) confused and depressed and unaware that menopause could be the cause of their insomnia, depression, anxiety, lack of sex drive, weight gain, mood swings - feeling empty and angry and alone. Worrying about, or recovering from a broken relationship, feeling the rage, feeling something was just "wrong" with them.   After many such conversations, I felt a strong drive to try and do something more than just learn other women's stories, I knew I should share them so perhaps I could help other women know they weren't alone in what they were going through.

I don't know that woman's name. I wish I did.   She's the real reason I wrote this book and I owe her a true debt of gratitude for her opening up and sharing her true feelings.

❧

PART 2.

IN THESE PAGES:
THE PROCESS & THE INTENTION

The stories you are about to read were gathered in a variety of ways. My initial work on this project began in the days just a few months prior to the onset of the pandemic, back when it was still ok to meet face to face. Most of those interviews are with people I know - friends, relatives, colleagues.

Once lockdown came about, I switched tracks and started a social media page to encourage women to share their story for the project. I was really encouraged by the feedback and support from the social media group, so I began joining every online forum and chat I could find on the topic, virtually reaching out and asking participants to consider sharing their stories as well. The response was incredible!! I've scoured the internet for firsthand accounts from all over the globe, from magazines, blog sites, women's health forums - anywhere I could find a real life story or experience.

I am continually encouraged to see many more notable public figures are coming forward to openly discuss their menopause experiences, and have included some excerpts from their previously published stories and interviews.

The result is this collection containing a wide spectrum of real life, firsthand accounts, designed to give women the unique experience of sharing with a vast collective of unique women from all walks of life. Real life stories that describe in depth what menopause actually FEELS LIKE, what helped and what didn't, and for those who have "crossed over" what their life is like now.

There is no hidden agenda or position intended from this book. All opinions hold equal weight here, and all strategies are valid. We are all unique individuals, and different things work for different people.

This book is not intended to provide medical advice, but rather to give the reader context and exposure to a range of menopause realities, to broaden the knowledge base of the reader. Think of it as a tribal circle in which we are sharing our personal histories to teach the next generation.

Sit with this book and absorb the stories as they were intended. Each one is someone's personal truth, their daily reality. While not everything will resonate with your situation, there is value in gaining perspective on the wide spectrum of experiences that exist. As they say, knowledge is power.

I wish that every reader finds a little piece of themselves or someone they know in these pages, and are comforted knowing they are not alone.

This is the book I was looking for, but couldn't find on the shelf. My greatest hope is that these stories are helpful & that this book will be one that is shared and re-shared in your personal circle with those you love and care for...... your sisters, your daughters, your friends.

PART 3
SHORT SUM UPS

SOME PEOPLE JUST HAVE A WAY OF EXPRESSING THEMSELVES SO WELL IN JUST A FEW SHORT WORDS. LET'S DIVE IN TO THE RANGE OF EXPERIENCES!

Jo's Story, Age 56

Several years ago my periods started to stutter, with a few six week gaps. The worse thing was that my moods were no longer predictable. The energy expended to keep myself civil was exhausting.

A couple of years on, the hearing in my right ear declined and I developed tinnitus. I started waking up at the dreaded 3am with a racing heart and mind, unable to get back to sleep. I also started to suffer waves of inflammation where my whole body would ache for hours, then days, and sometimes weeks on end.

I was really cranky and unsettled at work - my 30 year career in environment and sustainability was always challenging and rewarding, but my well of patience and diplomacy had run dry. At the instigation of some caring friends and my partner, I took all my long service leave, bought a welder and taught myself to weld from YouTube.

But then the waves of inflammation and fatigue got worse, and became my permanent existence. I was losing words and concepts, and found making decisions excruciating - I thought I was suffering early onset dementia.

After holding out for so long, I decided to try MHT/HRT, hopeful that it may help and bracing myself for disappointment. It's been a life changer for me. A year after Menopausal Hormone Therapy, I am back working on a large public sculpture, running a kilometer every morning, and keeping up (kind of) with chores on our small holding. Life is good. ■

Melissa's Story, Age 52

I believe I went into perimenopause in my very early 40s. My periods stayed regular, but then slowly, I'd be woken most nights needing to pee. Then it became every night, for years. I'd get migraines every month for years and years. Always felt it was hormonal in my gut instinct, but no professionals ever asked about monthly cycles.

Moods, anxiety, forgetfulness all crept in. I'd had a doctor asking me if I was depressed, and offering me a script to help with it.

My libido took a long vacation, brain fog was horrible, sadness was awful, despite being happily married and getting the job I wanted and I was besotted with our new puppy. I discovered (the Menopause and Perimenopause Australia Facebook group), watched an *Insight* episode on menopause and the penny finally dropped. I found a women's health GP and she gave me MHT based on my symptoms. Two years down the track, I'm happy, calm, able to recall details, although the libido is still absent, I'm at least not moody. ■

Lily's Story, Age 45

My perimenopause started well before I even knew what it was, at around 39. My libido went crazy, I was like a wild animal, and as a newly single woman I was killing it. It was the time of my life, but the honeymoon did not last.

After the high came the low, and then the lower, and then an even lower low until I felt like I had completely lost my sense of self and my place in the world. It is a difficult thing to explain, but an impossible feeling to live with. I wasn't me.

When I looked in the mirror, I was ageing before my eyes, well before my time. I felt so alone.

Then after 4 years of personal investigation, all on my own, I discovered what perimenopause was. It was a revelation and a glint of hope.

I'm a long way from where I want to be; the strong, fit, vibrant and alive woman I know is still in there; but I can see her now, and I know I'll find her again soon. ■

Lisa's Story, Age 52

I feel so lucky. I managed to fall pregnant at 44 and the following year I started peri, with my periods becoming more and more erratic. I'm now menopausal and to be honest, I've not found it too bad. I had lots of hot flushes during peri and I still have body sweats at night, but they are gradually getting better. I do have more digestive issues and things I used to love like curry, no longer love me.

I suffer from insomnia and usually get by on four hours sleep, waking at 2ish most mornings. At first, I used to get distressed by it, but now I try to look at it more positively… I see it as a bit of me time when I read or Google weird things. I also have zero problems with my sex drive. In fact, there has been little to no change in that respect. ■

Tammy's Story, 39

I went into surgical menopause at 36 years old, post-hysterectomy and having my ovaries removed. All of the menopause symptoms hit all at once, hot flushes, body aches, mood swings, loss of libido, insomnia…

Then I had to navigate the world of HRT. My surgeon had no idea, my GP even less… There is still so much fear around HRT. I was scared to say I needed it. I received ridiculous advice from friends telling me HRT would kill me…

Also, all of the menopause pamphlets feature women in their late 50s. I felt so alone. No one looked like me. I couldn't identify with anyone and I felt so out of place.

Now I'm on the right path. I will probably need medication until I'm 50. So another 10+ years but I don't care because after nearly three years, I'm starting to get my life back. ■

Elaine's Story, Age 52

My experience has been pretty tame with perimenopause so far - the odd occasional hot flush which is a very strange sensation. Aside from that, I haven't had any other issues with it. I think I have been very lucky but my mum didn't have much of an issue with it either. ■

Melinda's Story, Age 48

Ugh. Where to start? My symptoms probably started two years ago. The hot flushes that feel like someone has put you in a furnace; these can cause an intense feeling of panic.

The all-over itchiness, that feels like a million bugs running just under the surface of your skin (also known as formication). For me, formication always hits at night just when I'm in that sleepy sweet spot. Many nights I have put the lights on just to check I'm not actually covered in bugs.

The feeling that my body (and mind) isn't my own; aches and pains, brain fog, dizziness, bladder issues. The distance between my partner and I because, firstly I'm snappy, irritable and overly sensitive and secondly because I have zero desire to even be touched, let alone have sex. ■

Amanda's Story, Age 44

I experienced sudden onset chronic migraines at 37. I went through every grueling migraine prophylactic medication out there.

Just after turning 42, I found a significant and relentless increase in my migraine severity, in combination with forgetting simple things I wouldn't normally. Then my eyes needed eye drops daily and my mouth felt like it was on fire. I started to experience hot flushes, vaginal atrophy, and what felt like PMS all the time.

I requested a referral to an endocrinologist. During the wait, I started experiencing entire days in bed unable to stop crying, I'd never experienced depression before. I was suicidal, and it happened so fast. My anxiety was off the charts. I was very fortunate to have a partner to get me to appointments and make sure I was okay.

My endocrinologist diagnosed me almost straight away based on my obvious symptoms. MHT has helped significantly with my hot flushes, skin and hair health and vaginal symptoms, but it wasn't until my dose was quite high that I felt a sense of well-being that had been missing the whole time. Unfortunately, that is not always around, and I've had to start antidepressants too. I'm still just waiting out this hard time.

My endocrinologist has been very realistic regarding expectations, and that perimenopause will just be hard for me. I'm in the severe spectrum of symptoms.

I am definitely doing better than I was, but it's hard work. ■

Catherine's Story, Age 51

I've just had one year of no periods today. I haven't had any hot flushes or side effects of any note. I have given up alcohol (previously a lifelong huge drinker) and have just lost nearly 20kg.

My mental health and clarity has improved and I feel better physically and mentally than I have in my entire life. I'm waiting to see now after 12 months no period if suddenly my side effects are going to come at me hard and fast! I've spent a year or more waiting and wondering... is this it? ■

Kim's Story, Age 61

I'd heard women talk about menopause, but mostly it was hot flashes and night sweats. I never experienced them. What I didn't know was that perimenopause was going to be a difficult time.

I had two periods a month. No one had ever said that was a possibility. I went to my gynecologist and said "Is something wrong?" She said, "No, this is normal for many women." At the time, I felt completely out of sorts. It was the first time I ever experienced depression.

Oh, and the hair loss! Everyone always thought I had very thick hair but instead I had a lot of very thin hair. Anyway, it thinned out to a level that my parents thought I had some dread disease. I happened to see a tiny article in the paper where doctors at a nearby hospital were experimenting with a drug to help women with menopausal hair loss. It worked.

Post menopause I have few issues. Moods levelled when I quit having periods. And oh, it's so great not having periods! The drugs help me keep my hair! It's still a bit thin, but so much better than it could be. The chin hair is a problem, but I just tweeze them or wax them from time to time. ■

Cindy's Story, Age 64

I'm nearly 10 years past menopause. It takes more exercise to keep the fat off but I've got more time to do that now. Same with libido - you have to deliberately preserve and maintain.

Menopause was pretty mild for me, really. My sleep got worse - alcohol hurts, exercise helps - but mostly I'm much happier and more comfortable with being my authentic self now that I'm not controlled by hormones. I'm more in control.

If you're willing to take responsibility for your own health, post-menopause can be more fulfilling than you might imagine. Younger women tend to understand the importance of self-care now and that gives them a big advantage. ■

Ann Fletcher's Story, Age 54

A team leader for a specialist homelessness service in Newcastle, had been dealing with mild perimenopausal symptoms since her mid-forties. It ramped up in 2020 when she suddenly became so lethargic she could barely stay awake while driving her car.

"I had been a fit and active person and suddenly I had zero energy," Fletcher says. "Initially, I put it down to the fact we were in a pandemic and I had my kids and grandkids all living with me. I wasn't getting a lot of sleep! But after watching an episode of the SBS show *Insight* about menopause and joining an online community group of women on Facebook, I knew there must be more to my lethargy."

Ann completed the Australasian Menopause Society's 'symptom checker' questionnaire and took the results to her GP. After further investigations, she was prescribed Menopausal Hormone Therapy MHT (previously known as HRT) and within 10 days, Ann says her life was transformed.

"I got my energy back and began sleeping better and the hot flushes disappeared. While I know everyone is different, the hormone treatment was remarkably effective for me." ■

Siobhan's Story

It was a surprise for Siobhan when she experienced the first signs of menopause at 35. She had no family history of early menopause and had not had any surgery that might bring it on.

I was 35 and going through a bad time with very heavy periods, which never seemed to end. I was having dreadful night sweats; I was up 5 or 6 times a night. I also had uncontrolled hot flushes at work during the day. My moods were very erratic and my temper was wild – I'd fly off the handle for no reason. I really didn't know what was going on with me at the time. I thought I was just finding life extra hard. I felt out of control and very lacking in confidence to make decisions, which made my temper all the worse. Eventually, I was diagnosed as having early menopause.

It was a total shock. Because now I knew, I definitely couldn't have children. This was devastating news, as I hadn't had children. And I got the news at a time when all the talk among my friends was of how so many women were having babies into their 40s. I wanted children, I really love children, I work with children. I have three nieces who I absolutely adore, but would love to have had my own. This confirmation of the fact that I couldn't have any children of my own was very, very hard to accept.

Having the diagnosis of premature menopause gave me an explanation, which was very, very helpful. At least knowing that it was the menopause gave it a name and made me realize that I wasn't just going mad. I was given HRT, mainly because my night sweats were so bad and it also helped with my temper. I'd advise others to find out all about HRT because there is a lot of new information out there.

I managed to get over it, with a lot of work, once I realized what I was going through. I think you need to get treatment and help and then get on with your life as soon as possible. ■

Maria's Story

I always thought that the menopause happened to women in their 50s which seemed a lifetime away when I was in my early 40s. I was even more surprised when I started to get the odd hot flush in my 40s but since then and in the last number of years it has taken over my life. Nobody talks about the night sweats, the sleepless nights not to mention the mood swings and it's this that I find hard to come to terms with. At present I'm keeping positive by doing yoga and meditating as we'll as having had some homeopathy but everyone is different and we all need to find what works best for us. ■

Dee's Story

I only started experiencing any type of symptoms last year, at age 49. I got hot flushes at night and so couldn't sleep. It was driving me crazy; I kept turning the fan on and off all of last summer. My periods are only just beginning to go a bit weird now – one this month, none last month – it's going like that.

I knew it was coming. I've had a workmate who's been going through it for a long time. As well as that, I remember my mum going through menopause. I have a vivid memory of my mother fainting from a powerful hot flush when I was about 13. That freaked me out, but for me, it's only really a night time thing. Mum experienced menopause early – in her early 40s. I think she said it was all done and dusted for her by the time she was 44.

There are girls at work who are at this time of their life, too. We talk about menopause a lot – we're pretty open there. I work with a broad range of ages, both young and old, so it's pretty cool.

It was the non-sleeping that really got me – I was turning into a grumpy old tart! ■

Hannah B's Story

This is completely out of my comfort zone and I've debated back and forth about whether to write about this, but I think it's really important to raise awareness about a very unspoken subject and it may help someone else.
At the beginning of the year, I decided to give my body a break and come off the pill for a bit. 10 weeks later no regular cycle and hadn't been feeling myself; feeling low, really anxious, memory fog, hot flushes, and noticed changes in my body.
Multiple scans and blood tests later I find out it's premature menopause. With no exact reason as to what causes it, but this affects 1 in 1,000 women under 30. I also received my AMH level, 0.05 = very low fertility/undetectable.. at the age of 28 this is not the result you expect. Shocked has been an understatement but I am mainly annoyed that no one talks about this whole subject and just assume that your body is working like everyone else's because of the constant pregnancy posts on social media. I eventually found a wonderful doctor who prescribed me HRT and after 2.5 weeks I suddenly felt like myself again! I know there is such a bad reputation around HRT but I did so much research and have discovered how vital it is for your own health and wellbeing. ■

Bobbins059 Story

I'm 55 & everything has been getting worse over the last 18months since giving up smoking but through my forties periods starting changing, I haven't had a period for about 11 months now. I've read many forums regarding the "the change" & found that I'm not the only one going through hell. These weird body sensations, feelings of low blood sugar etc & the anxiety, spikes in blood pressure OMG is it ever going to end, everything I do or don't do is dependent on how I feel, I'm almost now housebound, just when I think I might feel normal(sort of) & go out this wave of scary sensations come over me...I have to eat, I have to go home, I end up in a pool of crazy tears. Because of family history HRT is out also to as I take blood pressure meds. My Doc says it's all hormones, my blood tests have always been normal, I'm taking Vitamin B complex & have tried magnesium....aaarrgggh I want this to end, feels like this is going to take me out! Thanks ladies for 'listening' to my woes. ■

Anonymous Story

This is more of a rant so I can feel better but is it just me or has perimenopause/menopause changed and ruined your life? Life as I once knew it will never be the same, I feel like I'm living in purgatory day after day....leading in to year after year, every month seems to keep getting worse! This horrible journey began for me 6 years ago when I was still in my 30s, I would pray every week that things would get better or after my period went away I would feel a little better...I can say this I haven't seen a period in over 200 days and I feel worse! Over the years I have tried antidepressants (made things worse) tried hormones (made things worse) tried eating a little better (didn't notice any difference), tried vitamins with no change, tried probiotic and noticed no difference.....I have even been in counseling for 5 years in case its "all in my head".....nothing has helped me. My days now consist of waking up every morning not wanting to get out of bed, I drag myself to my bathroom to take my bath, I look in the mirror and see a bony sick lady who looks twice her age staring back at me. I try to force myself to eat throughout the day (I'm lucky if I get 4 bites in me), then for the next 12 hours I fight nausea and lower gut gurgling while the food attempts to digest, I feel tired and so depressed, I can't go any place or else my anxiety explodes, I can't feel happy about anything cause my stomach hurts, my head hurts, I feel lightheaded/dizzy, I have a ringing in my ears, I have lost most of my sense of taste, I have NO sex drive, I have facial twitches that I had never had before in my life, insomnia at times, my skin and hair are so dry nothing helps it.....and after having several medical tests the doctor tells me "You are a completely healthy woman"! This is not healthy and I feel as though menopause has taken so much from me. I feel like I'm in the movie groundhog day where I'm reliving the same nightmarish day over and over, nothing is changing! I am so sorry all of you strong women have to suffer with this same problem as I do....they should label it a disease not a transition! ■

The following section are anonymous candid comments from American women when asked to give their thoughts on menopause……share anything you'd like about your menopause was the question…..and here we go!!!!

"What really got me is when the hot flashes got to the point when you're standing in front of a customer and all of a sudden you start to drip sweat, and nobody says anything." ■

"For me, it's more of a marker of stepping into the next phase. It's more of a philosophical place where my energy is going and not so much coping with physical changes." ■

"It was being set free from buying all the sanitary towels all those years, and without having the pain of a period. Absolutely worth it. Absolutely worth it." ■

"So, I think society wise, it's very, very difficult, because you don't really know who to talk to, and most people don't really want to talk about it, even in talking with some people about, 'hey, I think I'm going to do this podcast. It sounds like a great opportunity' they'd be, 'why do you want to do that? Why do you want to expose yourself,' and I'm thinking expose myself to what? And at that, that is, I think the barrier, the barrier has to do with kind of, ignorance." ■

"Eventually, I started realizing, oh, I need to ask other people, maybe they can give me ideas of what they do. I remember asking a co-worker and she told me, you know what she said what I do when I feel it coming on, I put my wrists under the water. And that seems to cool me down. So, I tried that and I don't know it, it seemed to work sometimes and then at other times, it didn't work, but it was still worth a try. And gosh, then I did ask somebody else and they said you know at all times, make sure you have a fan. And so, I bought certain fans whenever I would get somewhere and they have fans, I always have fans everywhere." ■

"Then I started noticing that if I kept still and just kept still and quiet and let it come, and then it would go away, I would feel better. So, once I did that, and as soon as it started coming on, I just stayed calm. Then it would come on, and then it would leave." ■

"Then the next thing that helped me personally was somebody telling me that when they would ease up on their sugar, instead of eating a lot of sweets and sugar, they felt much better. So I said, okay, there's no harm. Let me scale back on the sugar. And that seemed to help me, not saying that they went away, but they became better and less intense. But I must say that the time, the night sweats went away for me totally. And I haven't had them since was me, really making sure that I work out at least three to four times a week; walking, nothing vigorous, but absolutely put in time in workout. When I do that, I don't get them at all. And the moment I stop, if I stop for a week, and I haven't done any workout, they come on strong. So for me, it's my inspiration to really work out so that works for me." ■

"After the hot flashes, and then you're not sleeping and then your body starts changing. A great example is my husband at one point was like, 'do you have to always have these hot flashes?' And I'm like, I have absolutely no control over hot flashes. So, I ended up giving him a commentary for a day. So, every time that I had a hot flash, I would say, I'm having one. I'm having one. By about mid-afternoon he finally said, okay, I get it, you're having them a lot. And I think that was something that if I hadn't have actually told him initially, and done that commentary with him, it would have been something again, that I would have just taken on that, you know, I'm the only one that's having to go through this and I'm going to fight it on my own." ■

"I was working really hard on not minimizing or invalidating my concerns, and my disappointments and my complaints. You know, we, we do that to women a lot, you know, we say, 'oh, she's on the rag', 'oh, you must be expecting your period'. You know, and we'll dismiss ourselves you know, 'I'm sorry for being so emotional, I'm premenstrual', we dismiss our minds and our emotions and our reactions and responses to the world based on our hormones, and I was trying not to do that. I wanted to figure out can I separate; you know how much is exacerbated because I know what I'm feeling is valid. And I don't want anyone to say, you know, you're acting like a crazy menopausal person, because then the rage would really take over and the badassery would really come out and I'd have to be really mean to someone." ■

"I don't remember the onset of the rage. I just remember being very angry a lot of the time when I was in the house, feeling unhappy a lot of the time when I was out of the house, and being very quick to be triggered to the rage." ■

"So early on, when I first exhibited the menopausal symptoms, I certainly had mood changes and mood swings. So, when I first started going through the mood changes, I didn't really know what was happening and certainly my, my two daughters did not know what was happening. So, they, they made me these little symbols, which I have in my hand, one's a smiley face one's a frown face. And the bottom bracket says mood with a colon, and so what they invited me gently, kindly and lovingly to do is when I was in a good mood to give them a little fair warning, and show the smiley face and when I was not in a good mood to just show the frowny face so that they could steer clear, and everybody would be happy and well adjusted. And I found, just like, with most things in life, if you bring the people who are closest to you in to what's happening, and you talk about it, and you communicate about it, it's so much easier, as opposed to trying to hide what's happening or be embarrassed about it. You know, it just ends up making it harder on everybody." ■

"One of the other symptoms that I probably didn't really mention much was the, the anxiety that I would feel and knowing that I couldn't say anything, I would feel it was, was like knots in your stomach and, and I don't know your hands would sweat like the normal feelings of anxiety is like, I-don't-want-to-do-it-have-to-do-it-but-I don't-want-to-do-it. I don't. I don't want to go to work. I want to stay home, and I want to stay away from people because they don't understand, and I want to talk to someone. But they're not there. And sometimes I felt emotional. I felt as though I wanted to cry, and I didn't have really a reason to cry. Or, I thought I didn't have a reason to cry. But when I think back, I did have reasons to cry." ■

"Going through menopause quietly wasn't easy. What I realized that I had to do was I had to find answers to why I was feeling the way that I was feeling. And I did a lot of research cause you can Google anything these days, and I would, I would Google symptoms of menopause, menopause, I would Google, how to handle, how to how to walk through, through life with this, how to talk about it, what you can say to start a conversation. I did a lot of research on each of the symptoms that I was going through to get an answer. I had a better understanding when I did research. So, during my research, I learned that there are things that you can do to help you to manage your emotions. I read about meditation and sitting still and actually breathing, and that would help." ■

"What I did find for myself is that even though I was having all these physical changes, I also had the emotional kind of where I was having just crazy anxiety that was coming out of nowhere, at that point, then had some tools that I was able to utilize with, you know, deep breathing, I was using some yoga. The other thing that I did in the midst of all of this is, I also added in doing even more formal meditation and I'm glad that I actually started that earlier, much earlier than when I was in the crux, and the worst part." ■

"All my physicians have been the same physicians I've had for years. The reason I do that is because I want to cultivate a relationship with my physician, that, especially as I'm aging, that's one of the most important relationships I'm going to have, is with my physician. And so if I have a relationship with them where I'm able to be open to them, and then even find out more about who they are as a person as opposed to just a physician, that builds trust, once it builds trust, then you know, that physician has your best interest at heart. And then you are also able to be open. And so because I'm that way, I always insist that I get to know the physician first. Before they treat me before anything, I have to sit down with them, tell them who I am and I ask them who they are, on a personal level, as much as they willing, and able to tell me all about themselves. After I create that relationship, and then they built that trust, then you will find that, in fact, I insist on having appointments where the doctor has more time, whether it's early in the morning does the first patient or late the last patient, because I really want them to spend time with me. And that has worked out brilliantly for me really has. And I do love my physicians I really do." ∎

"Well, I can imagine the kind of conversations I would have to have with someone new. In my mind, I'm very open and straightforward and brave, in order to say, here's what's going on with me at this time in my life, and if we become sexual, this is what I'm gonna need from you. I think the conversation would have to be very explicit. Some things that are easier to say like, intimacy is not the same as intercourse. So, a lot of physical intimacy, arousal can take longer. So, we may have to talk about more foreplay. I would need to make sure that any partner–I'm stealing this line from someone–but that any partner was not 'illcliterate', that they were aware of female genital geography. And I would have to be very open and clear about what I needed from myself and from the partner and that person would have to be very patient and responsive in the moment because sometimes that means stopping or changing or slowing down." ∎

"I am describing a considerate lover but more importantly, I'm describing being a person who tells what will hopefully be a considerate lover, what she needs. You can have a considerate lover and never open your mouth and still not get your needs met. You know. So, it's more about that two-way street and I think that would have to be initiated by me, you know, I'm sure male sexuality changes with age as well. And women throughout their whole life, I think we should be talking to our partners much more throughout our whole life. But I think it's truly, truly vital after menopause, because things work vastly differently." ∎

"The beauty for me was that I have, my sister is great. And so the laughter of being … we're very close in age. We were on the similar paths, and being able to talk to her and laugh about some of the things that we were going through and kind of just find humor in it, I think really helped to kind of ease the, the anxiety and the stress of it. I think that was very helpful. I will say it would have been nice to have more of a pack that you could go to where you didn't feel like it was only you know, a family or your very, very closest friends." ∎

"And I think that's something that, that women, the more we talk about it, the more we come out and, you know, bond, come together and realize, hey, we're all in this together, then the more opportunities that we're gonna be able to break those barriers and break down those fences that have been placed before us, where we do feel like we're isolated or that we cannot talk or that we have a much harder time finding, quote, kind of that pack, our pack. You know, those people that we can bond together with." ■

Marigarcia123's Story

I am 57 years old. I started peri menopause 5 years ego. I had a horrible perimenopause. Horrible sinuses, I felt extremely anxiety with horrible panic attacks, and servers .constipation I would wake up every day with doom & gloom feelings, I felt dizzy every day and felt like I walked unsteady (even now) after two years of post menopause. Now I am experiencing walking up feeling emotionally drain and "down" feelings. I experienced anger during my perimenopause. I am not an angry by nature so I knew this has something to do with hormones going hay wired. I felt so overwhelmed sometimes I didn't know what to do with myself. I called people that had offended me trough the

years because I felt the need to clear the air and felt it very therapeutic. I wasn't able to deal with stress like I did all my life now but wasn't able to handle a fork falling of a table before it felt like World war 3!

Now post menopause (two years after) and I feel like I am back to perimenopause with horrible mental specially feelings. My life has been and absolute hell since all of this started. I walked every day and worked for years under a lot of stress I am super happy in my marriage and my life is a lot not stressful. So yes, my menopause experience has been truly a life changing experience. Don't wish any of this on my worst enemy. ■

❦

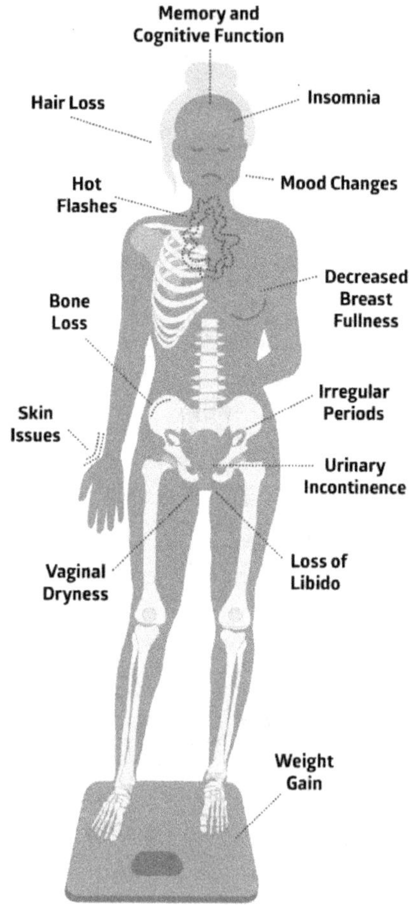

The 13 Most Common Menopause Signs and Symptoms
Memory and Cognitive Function
Hair Loss
Insomnia
Hot Flashes
Mood Changes
Bone Loss
Decreased Breast Fullness
Skin Issues
Irregular Periods
Urinary Incontinence
Vaginal Dryness
Loss of Libido
Weight Gain

PART 4
QUICK READS

DEEPER IN DETAIL, THESE STORIES RUN A PAGE OR TWO FOR WHEN YOU HAVE A LITTLE EXTRA MOMENT…….

Shelley's Story

I'm Shelley, I share my time between Cornwall and Norfolk in the UK, I'm 46 years old. I've been a stay at home mum for the last 18 years and Director of my son's Ltd Company for the last 10 years! I have been a Learning Disabilities nurse and carer for others most of my life, we were a Foster family when I was nine years old. Taking care of others and putting others first is what has impacted my current health circumstances and challenges. I didn't do any 'self-care' when I needed to.

I'm still perimenopausal, signs of that started showing up in 2015, 4 years ago, but I get the whole spectrum of menopausal symptoms plus the heavy flooding!

I was able to research a lot of my symptoms, other than that I don't mention them much, unless in the company of other women! I think it's healthy to share issues. However, my journey and recovery from PTSD over the last 6 months has been really quite dramatic and successful and I now really want to share my story of recovery to inspire other women and to educate women who have experienced trauma in early life or teens that PTSD is a risk factor in Perimenopause.

Hair loss, anxiety, loss of muscle tone were symptoms I initially experienced, followed by three years of depression and a PTSD diagnosis

2018. Flooding became a huge problem three years ago rendering me housebound for 3 days and often needing to change clothing half-hourly. Premenstrual symptoms have been awful with tender breast, emotional ups, and downs. My main reason for completing this questionnaire is to share my PTSD recovery story without NHS support/counselling. Symptoms that have subsided with supplements include night sweats and hot flashes, emotional up, and downs, tearful mornings, I'm still easily brought to tears but in appropriate situations!! Cravings for carbs, anxiety. Agoraphobia.

 I've tried to do things as naturally as I can avoiding mainstream interventions as much as possible, I've found www.wellsprings-health.com to be an invaluable source of information on the hormonal challenges and found their natural Progesterone cream to be hugely beneficial. I also take their Menopause supplement. I completed a BSc in Nutritional Medicine whilst bringing up my children, qualifying just as my son's Company took off, so although I've benefitted from that injection of nutritional knowledge, I've had little opportunity to share it with others. ◼

Robyn's Story

I have to say for an educated, fairly worldly wise person, I was quite shocked and a little bit devastated. Having experienced days of strange feelings, thundering heart beats and aches and pains where I shouldn't have them, at least now I had an answer. In a way I was relieved.   At least I am not dying but I did officially acknowledge to my ovaries that their work here was done. They had given me 4 beautiful children who I fully intend driving nuts in my old age! I was so frightened though. I really thought something very ominous was happening and as I have more than once before sought out an explanation, I say again, thank god for Wikipedia!

Menopause! It's a natural process and once I embrace it, I will be fine.

What is strange though, is the fact that women don't talk about it.....really. They talk about everything else but women do not generally like discussing this event even though it occurs over a 2 to 3-year period. If anything, it's a topic that generates laughter rather than frank discussion. It's not something they want to admit to each other and it surprises me that being such an information junkie that I know so little about it.

It's a process that happens over a period of time and can affect women in various ways. For me, the aches and pains, weight gain along with the mood swings was a dead giveaway. Despite being told by the GP that I was a little young, I went on the sage advice of my mother who told me that she had started around the same age. I was tempted to try HRT to see if that would help but not being too fond of artificial drug therapy I resisted the urge.

And as for my libido, well that's gone down the pan now. When I was thirty something, having a husband seven years younger than me was fantastic but now, not being on the same hymn sheet so to speak can cause some inevitable problems!

I just needed to make some small lifestyle changes like cutting down on the carbs and increasing my vegetable and fruit intake. It's hard to know whether I am getting the hot flush symptom as living in New Zealand, the weather here is quite warm and having worked with a friend who suffered from hot flushes, it's a symptom I am glad that I do not have.

I am hoping with time; I grow more relaxed with my new self. However, I find that I just can't stand looking at my reflection or pictures of myself and at times, I grieve for the person that seems to have disappeared fairly suddenly. Surely there is an upside? I will have to wait and see!

AND I AM NOT GIVING UP MY COFFEE IN THE MORNING! ◼

Dana's Story

I was unceremoniously plunged into menopause when I was diagnosed with breast cancer last year. In addition to having to cope with starting chemotherapy, losing all my hair and also losing a breast, I was subject to horrible hot flushes. They were very intense at first, and would inevitably happen just as I was falling asleep. I would suddenly be uncomfortably hot and prickly and drenched in sweat. So I would throw off the duvet, and my pyjamas and the beanie I was wearing to keep my bald head warm and wait to cool down, until I could sleep for an hour or two before waking up yet again, drenched in sweat. So for the months that I was undergoing treatment, I had very little quality sleep.

The hot flushes happened during the day as well. I remember how, as a child, I would laugh at women fanning themselves with sheaves of paper, and then that was me, at the dinner table, in the synagogue, while chatting to my friends. I would be desperately trying to coax a breeze from whatever piece of paper was available.

It was unpleasant, but I consider myself fortunate in that the symptoms were manageable and lessened a little over time. I never had to explore treatment for the symptoms. But more importantly I was nearly 50 when I was diagnosed and began my chemotherapy. I would have been menopausal anyway. In the months that I was receiving treatment at the oncology centre I met several women in their 30's and 40's and even one woman in her 20's who were menopausal as a result of their chemotherapy treatment. For these younger women the transition was premature and deeply painful.

Many of the female cancers are hormone driven. This means that women who have had breast cancer or ovarian cancer cannot be treated with hormone replacement treatment. Even natural hormones and many herbal remedies are not considered to be altogether safe as they may feed the cancerous cells. Low doses of SSRI's (anti-depressants) are apparently effective in managing hot flushes, but do little to improve the mood swings and anxieties that often accompany menopause. For cancer survivors the best hope seems to be a combination of counseling, and biofeedback training to manage the emotional and physical fall out of menopause. ■

Ati's Story

Ati, an integrative wellbeing therapist was in her forties when she underwent an urgent hysterectomy. She had a long history of endometriosis and adenomyosis, which had left her in excruciating pain from heavy periods and uterine fibroids. The hysterectomy meant that she lost all of her estrogen overnight which put her into an immediate state of surgical menopause.

One week after she had her hysterectomy, Ati was hit with the distressing news that she had life-threatening blood clots in both of her lungs. Thankfully, she battled through, and overcoming these huge blows to her personal health made Ati confident she could survive anything.

The physical symptoms of Ati's menopause were much more challenging than the mental ones. "I had endless hot flushes. My body temperature was permanently completely freezing or burning hot and I was also experiencing unbearable night sweats. I had severe joint pain, started to lose my hair and had vaginal atrophy. But I was not going to let the menopause defeat me."

As a wellbeing therapist, who often supported menopausal women, she felt like she had the tools to be able to handle the effects on her mental health; however, some symptoms were much harder for her to deal with than others. "I had no idea of the extent of the changes my body would go through" she explained, "and if the body is depressed then the mind can follow suit very quickly."

Ati's mission in life changed as a result of her menopause. She now makes it her purpose as a wellbeing therapist to help others going through the menopause learn to cope through natural remedies, her personal favourites being essential oils, sage tablets, oral vitamin D spray and 'golden' turmeric lattes. She encourages her clients and other women and not be ashamed and to speak about what they are experiencing. ■

Karin's Story

I have no real idea when I started the menopause, I suppose like many women I realised one day that the things that were happening to my body were symptoms of the menopause or **perimenopause**. This did not upset me, in a way it was a relief as then I could begin to understand what was happening. The worst and most debilitating effect for me was torrential periods, I always had **heavy periods** from early on but things began to get problematic in my mid-thirties - (**early menopause**). Enough to say that there are crime scenes with less blood.

I had many of the other symptoms **mood swings, tiredness** and **weight gain,** and having suffered from migraines all my life they too got worse. So all in all, with two young children and a conglomerate of physical irritations I continued on with life thinking this is just how it is: getting older, stress of family life, work, money, relationships.

My approach was to attack each symptom individually, I took pain killers and other prescription drugs for my headaches and every available 'tonic' for the tiredness. Eventually after much I cajoling from my husband, I consulted a traditional **herbalist**. He gave me a tea to brew at home - it smelt and looked like 'Victorian drains'. It did help for a while, then other remedies and then something else. All worked for a short time but the effectiveness became less each time.

With the heavy bleeding it became almost impossible to leave the house during those few days of the month and I felt I needed something more effective and long lasting. My doctor suggested an IUD to inhibit the bleeding, I decided to go for it and yes it worked the bleeding stopped altogether! But all the other symptoms remained and as I got older they were joined by others - joint pain and the most telling of all the **Hot Flushes**.

I was getting fed up and eventually decided to try **HRT**. The symptoms eased but I hated it. I gained weight but mostly I felt that I had given up and in. I needed my body to be mine not run by artificial hormones. It was not for me I binned the patches.

What's Changed? My approach. I still have all these wonderful symptoms, what's changed is me. About eighteen months ago around the time of my HRT experiment, I began to think about how these symptoms were affecting my life and I came to an understanding that began to make sense to me. It is this, that the menopause and all the physical and psychological symptoms are within my power to control, I can react to them in a manner that works for me and makes my life better. All the therapies and medicines can help with the symptoms and some do, but it is my approach to the actual fact of the menopause that can make my life easier and more enjoyable.

I am not a psychologist, all I can say is that when I decided that I was not going to be controlled or overwhelmed by this stage in my life. That I was going to effectively consider it part of my everyday life, it did become easier. Yes, I have hot flushes, I wake at night (often) I feel tired, I feel irritable, I have joint pain, yes all of these! This is part of my life now and for the next while, so I live with it embrace it and get on with it. I don't take any medication, remedies or supplements for my menopausal symptoms! I take supplements for my overall health and the occasional pain killer for my headaches. I developed a new love for exercise which helps clear my mind and keep me positive.

So to say the menopause is in your mind is not to denigrate the very real symptoms that many women experience, me included. It is to help empower those experiencing symptoms both physical and psychological to overcome the debilitating effects of them and live happier easier lives. ■

Nicola's Story

Menopause was the last thing on my mind. Aged just 46 and beginning a new relationship, with my second novel hitting Number One on the Best Sellers List, life was good. I should have been on cloud nine. My dreams had all come true but I'd never felt more out of control. I had hit peri-menopause. My once excruciatingly painful, but regular periods became completely unpredictable. I began to experience two month gaps, then periods that were 4 week long with continuous bleeding. I was exhausted, weepy and terrified I was dying.

In the height of summer I could no longer wear light coloured dresses or plan a trip to the pool. Instead I had to wear dark jeans with long tops to cover me in case of a dreaded 'accident'. Not very ideal in the throes of a new relationship when I wanted to dress and impress. My decision to take my budding romance slowly was made easier by the fact that I had no desire to spend our first night together wearing pyjamas and two pads!

Normally a great sleeper, I began to wake around 3am, tossing and turning for hours resulting in my trying to get through the next day in an exhausted daze. I developed a metallic taste in my mouth which made me nauseous. I became intolerant to alcohol. Even one glass would send me to the porcelain bowl.

Dr. Google became my obsession. I suffered urinary frequency, bouts of cystitis. No wonder I was weepy!

After a night of lying on the bathroom floor simply as it was cool and close to the toilet I'd been throwing up in, after a night out and just one glass of wine, I decided that this was as bad as I wanted to get.

Wary of going on medication, I have taken the natural route of Aloe Vera gels, vitamins and gave up alcohol completely. I miss it, but for some reason my new peri-menopausal body simply could not tolerate it. I began to go to bed earlier, at around 9 or 10pm, so if I woke at 3am, which was for some reason my new 'wake up' time, I would at least have had a good few hours sleep. I gave up coffee after 6pm. I drank more water. I stopped googling every symptom and worrying that I had cancer. I accepted that my body is changing and acted accordingly.

I am kind to myself. I spent twenty-five years as a single Mum and both my kids have flown the nest. Now, I can put me first. If I need to have a nap, I will and if I need to stay in bed all day instead of doing housework, I will. I have not yet experienced hot flushes, or moodiness, or night sweats. Maybe they will come, hopefully not. I don't know what will be down the line for me - if the long-term bleeding will eventually stop as I reach the end of my menopausal years, or if I might need surgery sometime. I don't know if I will need HRT or pills. I do know that I have to accept this new stage of my life. It came upon me suddenly and knocked me for six – the realisation that I am 'middle aged and menopausal'! Yet, still I get the teenage girl butterflies of excitement when my new 'boyfriend' is picking me up for our date. Then when he tells me I look beautiful, I smile and thank him, clutching my handbag full of pads, painkillers, spare underwear and……. birth control. One has to be prepared for all possibilities! ∎

Karyn's Story, Age 49

I was diagnosed with breast cancer at age 39, and unfortunately, my treatment threw me into early menopause.

In some ways, it's a good thing I went through it then, because now I don't have to worry about things other women have to worry about. But at the time, I had hot flashes, my hair got really dry and thin, and my skin became dry and patchy. Because I didn't have many girlfriends going through it at the same time, I had a lot of questions. Luckily, I had a great team of doctors and some people in my cancer support groups who had been through it. And if I was hanging out with my mom and her friends and they were talking about it, I'd be like, "Yeah, I know what you mean!"

For me, the emotions associated with menopause probably fell under the same category of dealing with the changes that came from having breast cancer fairly young. I had a double mastectomy and went through menopause, so basically all the things that made me feel like a woman were eliminated at the same time. I felt like an old lady at 39.

At that age, I still had several friends who had babies and were <u>pregnant,</u> and I wasn't necessarily thinking that I never wanted any more kids. My husband and I had only been married a year, and prior to me getting cancer, we talked about having a child of our own (we both have kids from previous marriages). But all of a sudden, it just wasn't an option anymore. It was sad because it wasn't my choice; it was another repercussion of what I had been through. I believe everything happens for a reason, though.

People go through menopause differently, but for me, it wasn't as bad as I thought it would be. I got hot flashes, and it was weird, but not awful. It was kind of like when you got your first period as a preteen or teenager — it was a change, but it was just part of the continuum of life. You go through so many transitions in your life, from a girl to a teenager to a young adult to a mother…this is just another one.

I'm now the age most people hit menopause — around 51 is the average. Soon all my friends will be starting to join the club, and I'll be like, "Been there, done that." ◾

Michelle's Story, Age 53

For me, menopause started a couple of years ago. I'm not completely through it, but I think I'm through most of it. The symptoms I noticed were hot flashes, trouble sleeping and changes in physical appearance and mood. For me, hot flashes were the worst. I was in a constant state of hot flashes coming unexpectedly, and that was really frustrating and difficult.

All the women I know who have gone through menopause experienced something, even if it wasn't necessarily bad. From what I'd heard from my friends, I expected hot flashes to happen mostly at night and wake me up with night sweats. The reality for me was they would happen at any time of day or night, and they would come out of nowhere. They would start from the inside and move out, so that all of a sudden I would feel like the inside of my body was 120 degrees, and I couldn't stop it. It really felt like it was rising up like a thermometer. I would be sitting at dinner, sometimes with business colleagues at an event, and it would just start happening. In most of those situations, I tried to conceal it or would excuse myself and try to move to a cooler place or walk outside. But one time, and only once, I was having a hot flash in front of a complete stranger at a dinner, and I flat-out said, "I'm sorry, I'm having a hot flash." And she said, "I can actually see it."

I didn't talk to too many people about it — maybe just a couple of friends and my husband. My mother had had a partial hysterectomy when she was in her 30s, so I didn't experience watching her go through anything or get any hint of what I was going to go through. Most of my friends did not experience it the way that I did. I don't think it's a weird thing to talk about if you're talking to a woman, and I was never embarrassed about it, but I would not discuss it with a man other than my husband.

I actually read a book about it when I started going through it. Someone advised me to read it, but I found it completely useless. I just feel like it's something that's a rite of passage. You just have to allow your body to go through it. My best advice is to try your best to embrace it. Allow the process to take place. ■

Kim's Story, age 54

I felt like my menopause symptoms weren't that big of a deal because I had been through so much with my periods and endometriosis and fertility issues. I'd been through the ringer.

The worst part about menopause was that I went for about nine months without a period and thought it was over, but they tell you you're not really out of the woods until you go a full year [without menstruating]. I would get to nine or 10 months and then have a period, so it was like I was back to square one. That went on for about three years, where the periods were few and far between but never far enough to be able to say, "I'm done." But then, finally, it was over. It's been around two years now.

My periods were always bad, ever since a month before I had my first period at 16. I experienced painful cramping, nausea, diarrhea — all of that every month. The disorder I had was endometriosis, which causes pain and can interfere with fertility. I had to get a laparoscopy, a surgery used to diagnose and remove endometriosis, as well as a uterine polypectomy, a removal of small growths (polyps), twice.

Getting pregnant was really difficult for me. My daughter was kind of a fluke, born completely naturally with no help, but two years after she was born, we were trying again and nothing was happening. I went through various treatments, from low-intervention to extreme intervention, and I finally got pregnant with twins after my second attempt at in vitro fertilization. Pregnancy was what finally made all the period pain better for a while.

But after the twins were born, there was a point in my late 40s when I was having some very irregular flows — I think periods were coming every two weeks. It was hard to control it and plan around it. I considered getting a hysterectomy, but things were so busy with my life between family and work that I just didn't know how I could take time off to do the surgery. I didn't know which was worse — taking six months off to recover or dealing with the erratic periods. Ultimately, by procrastinating and not making a decision, the decision was made for me, and I dealt with it until it stopped. In hindsight, I think that irregularity was premenopausal.

When I finally went through menopause, I had some hot flashes, but they were really fast, only lasting a minute or two, and it was just a warm feeling. It wasn't annoying or aggravating or intrusive. I also started waking up at odd hours in the middle of the night, and I couldn't get back to sleep. Any emotional experiences I had probably came from a combination of the lack of sleep and the hormones. I think in total it lasted about a year. It's all relative, so because of the things I'd been through, I didn't think of it as a big deal.

I have a group of 14 girlfriends who all get together on a monthly basis, and menopause comes up sometimes. My friends are really funny and they joke about it while keeping tabs and taking notes. One friend had three important pieces of advice that everyone should hear: First, whatever you're going through, whether you think it may be unusual or not, talk about it with your doctors and other people. She was having blood clots the size of pancakes and had to get tested for anemia. Second, never feel embarrassed or inferior by whatever is happening. Some women feel hesitant talking about sexual components of it — getting your period all the time as a menopause effect isn't exactly romantic. You need that communication. Third, be open to Eastern medicine like acupuncture. That's what stopped her hot flashes. And if your doctor isn't willing to discuss those options, find a new doctor.

Talking to friends also puts your own experience in perspective. A couple of my friends did have hysterectomies, and several also had been through things like double mastectomies due to family histories of breast cancer or other major illnesses. I know some of those people went through harder things than I did.

Each woman's experience is different, but talking about it is good for everyone. ■

Jo's Story, Age 54

"I can't – I just can't do this anymore!" "I lean back against the shelves, drop my bags & start to sob. It's May 2013, I'm 48 and in Tesco's with my sons, then 16 & 12. I'm crying in the biscuit aisle, looking at the chocolate hobnobs and wondering how my life has come to this.

Anxious and overwhelmed, I'm desperate for a good night's sleep. Both my parents are going through chemotherapy & as a single working Mum I am holding on by my fingertips.

With hindsight, I realise I was experiencing the perimenopause, something I knew absolutely nothing about at the time.

I share the story with a friend who asks how much **exercise** I do. The answer is very little: holiday swimming, the odd aerobics class. She generously gives me an old rowing machine she no longer needs.

Within a couple of weeks of rowing in my kitchen, I am sleeping. Immediately I feel better & brighter. I join a gym, I no longer cry in supermarkets.

A few months later my Mum dies of lymphoma 4 days before Christmas. Our world is shattered. Curiously I find I'm still going to the gym, finding solace in the rowing machine whilst my heart breaks & breaks again.

A few months later, with no planning, I decide I'm going to raise money for Macmillan Cancer Support by rowing a million metres & marathon on the ergo. I row 10,000 m every other night for 8 months & on the 1st anniversary of Mum's death & 5 days before my 50th birthday, I row a marathon (26.2 miles).

By now I've been learning about the perimenopause & I realise that moving joyfully & regularly has a hugely beneficial effect on my wellbeing – physical, emotional & mental.

Having done barely any exercise for decades before that fateful day in 2013, I have returned to things I loved as a little girl. Body boarding, swimming in the sea, going for bike rides in the hills. I did Couch to 5k for the first time aged 52 & learned to surf at 53.

In August of this year, aged 54, I became the first woman to stand up paddleboard 162 miles coast to coast across the north, picking up litter & fundraising for The Wave Project & 2MinuteBeachClean community.

So what has the perimenopause given me?

- It forced me to start looking after myself after years of only looking after everyone else: early to bed, fresh air, moving joyfully, strength training, saying "no" more & being careful how I spend my energy & time.
- My tiny adventures in the sea & hills have helped me develop a much kinder relationship with my body & more positive body image.
- It's given me renewed purpose – fundraising for charity and picking up litter every day and on my PaddleboardTheNorth challenge.
- It's given me a voice. I am honoured to have been invited to share my story recently at Jane Dowling's Meno & Me menopause event about how exercise has helped me navigate the perimenopause. I hope I can show other women that they are not alone, they are not going crazy and there is hope ahead.

Passing on a message of hope & encouragement is perhaps the most special gift the menopause has given me. It makes all the times I cried in supermarkets worth it." ∎

Diane's Story, Age 47

"Today my 6 year old daughter Lola asked me what she could be when she was a 'Grown Up'. Sensing my opportunity to (not so) subtly push the 'Girls can Rule the World' mantra, I began my spiel about how she was going to have these amazing adventures and 'be whoever or whatever she wanted to be'.

"Maybe an astronaut" I suggested "Or a lawyer? An engineer, a teacher or. . ." She shook her head and interjected " . . . or a Rainbow Sparkle Fairy?"

A Rainbow Sparkle Fairy. Abso-freakin-lutely. Who the hell in their right mind would choose to be anything else giving the choice? I loved the certainty in her voice and the brilliantly, bat shit crazy world she inhabits, where this and pretty much anything and everything else is a possibility.

Conversely at 47 I am wading through the perimenopause and my own confidence and certitudes can get railroaded by fears of anxiety or self doubt. As my estrogen and the 'happy' hormones levels plummet my previous positive outlook can also take a nose dive. But at the risk of sounding #Blessed, witnessing Lola's wonderment while I explain why trees are simply amazing or seeing her mind being blown that we can turn corn kernels into actual popcorn, it's hard to maintain the melancholy. You get carried along by the excitement and newness of it all and remember 'y'know what —the world is a pretty awesome place'.

Having a small child keeps you very much grounded in the moment whereas midlife and in particular the onset of perimenopause can be a time of anxious reflection; looking to the past and dissecting the choices we've made or contemplating the future and the uncertainty of what happens next. The exhausting reality of dealing with a 6 year old bundle of snot, sass and silliness negates some of this hand wringing. I often feel I should be having a mid life crisis or at the very least some sort of perimenopausal panic. Maybe I am? but am too busy Googling 'how to do 'The Floss' or building a 'Café/Disco/Sleepover Hotel out of Lego to notice.

Don't get me wrong it's not all unicorns and glitter.

I worry that some of the negative physical and emotional effects of the perimenopause may impact on my ability to be good parent. I don't expect or aspire to be perfect but I sometimes fret that I am too 'shouty' as my tolerance levels and temper are significantly shorter these days. I get concerned that my erratic sleep means I often feel worn out and I don't have the same energy of the younger, non 'geriatric' mums.

Then there are times when I wistfully recall my younger 'London' days sans kids when I wore heels and drank white wine on sunny Saturday afternoons. Or look enviously at my friends who are either childfree or with grown up kids, as they plan their long weekends away or float about their (immaculate) homes lighting Diptyque candles in cashmere pyjamas.

Worst are the dark moments when I allow myself to think about the distant future. I am 4 decades older than Lola, she is an only child. I don't want her to be lonely or on her own. Ever. I agonise over becoming frail or ill. I don't want her to shoulder any burden of an aged parent. Ever.

But for now, to Lola, age is literally a (birthday) badge of honour and time is a concept she hasn't yet grasped. You are either a 'child', a 'grown up' or a 'wrinkly'. I currently reside in a subcategory of 'mum'.

She delights in counting my wrinkles "You haven't got that many, except these really, really big ones near your eyes' *sigh* and describes my ageing boobs as 'long' and 'flat' *sob*

Then – just when my self esteem is face down on the deck, she'll make me a card where she draws me with yellow hair and fabulous earrings and writes underneath 'To mummy, you are the bestest, most beautiful queen" *melt*.

These visceral emotional highs and lows are part and parcel of my experience of motherhood. Each morning I buckle up ready to withstand the emotional turbulence of the day ahead; Lola has the capacity to make my chest constrict with absolute love in one moment and then clench my knuckles with abject rage and frustration the next.

I am never sure if these erratic mood spikes are due to hormonal chaos or are just a by-product of being a parent. I expect we will find out when the menopause and puberty collide in a few years time (my husband is booking in his own midlife melt down for around the same time!). But in the meantime, in the here and now, this yellow haired 'Mummy Queen' is embracing every transient moment of this sparkly rainbow roller coaster ride." ■

Karen's Story

The last eighteen months have certainly been memorable. Feeling dizzy, off my food, and increasingly anxious, I gained the courage to talk it all over with a doctor, it transpired that I was anaemic, my blood pressure was high and I was peri-menopausal. A trio of trouble that was doing its best to chip away at my physical health and **mental well-being**.

Tiredness had seeped into all aspects of my life, acting like a domino effect on mood, rational thought, patience and ability to function day-to-day. Whilst in the midst of fitful sleep the early hours became familiar beasts to be slain: the midnight attempt to switch off, the 2am worries for the next day ahead, the 4am mental checklist to tick off, the 5am visit to the bathroom, the 6am acceptance that its almost time to get up anyway! With all that going on, it didn't occur to me that this tiredness was causing my low mood and crumbling of self-confidence.

I've always thought of myself as an organised person, in control, able to do many things and certainly more than capable of juggling work and home life and family commitments. All that came tumbling down, like the shifting walls of a sandcastle as the waves of daily demands washed over me. What was happening to me? With my former persona of being a strong woman came the unwritten rule that I didn't stop to tell anyone how I really felt anyway. I was too busy — there was always a job to be completed, something that I needed to do to help the kids or to support other relatives, a meeting or a deadline to meet for work.

When the tiredness and dizzy spells were at their worst, I think I broke. I felt like a cage was constructing itself around me, putting up barriers to hinder me from functioning as before. To put it succinctly, somewhere along the way I lost my confidence. Confidence can disappear in the blink of an eye but it takes so long to claw it back again to its former glory. I found myself doubting my abilities and questioning decisions that I had to make.

I had to take control. I started to write a blog and the responses I got opened my eyes: I was not alone. I re-evaluated my life and considered what positive measures I could take. I quit my long teaching career and am now writing, putting myself first when I can and achieved a long-held dream, publishing a book which tells my story – stumbling through motherhood, midlife and menopause. Writing has proved to be my therapy and asking for help and accepting support from family and friends, essential. I have been asked by a London media company to talk about my story, something that I find exciting and nerve-racking in equal measure but a definite privilege.

I am still struggling to break out of my confidence cage but I feel that I have located the key. ■

Kate's Story

For quite some time I've not felt like me – I fly off the handle at the tiniest of things, and the night sweats were out of control. Around February time I started to experience terrible heart palpitations and shortness of breath. I am awful at going to the doctors and tried to ignore it, however after a couple of panic attacks in March, as well as episodes of feeling very sad, low and uncontrollably angry, I felt I needed help, something I hate admitting.

Annoyingly, as we'd hit lockdown it meant I was unable to go to the doctor. I spent 3 months calling them every two weeks in tears and eventually after a rather desperate call I was sent for blood tests and a chest X-ray! Everything came back clear and having done much talking with experts I believe that what I am experiencing is perimenopause. Since I've acknowledged this, amongst other symptoms, the heart palpitations, breathlessness and panic attacks have decreased.

I still have moments of seeing red that can come from nowhere, which can have a huge impact on my family. But I am now under a consultant and hoping that I can get back to being 'me' soon. ■

Lisa's Story

I was around 46 or 47 when I started noticing **changes in my periods**. I was always regular, but now it was a complete blood bath! I had to work around my cycle because it got to a point where for 2 or 3 days I couldn't leave the house without flooding – no matter how many tampons/pads I was wearing. It was so uncomfortable and embarrassing – especially when I occasionally left stains on chairs and had to try and cover them up and rush off to get changed. My doctor suggested the Mirena coil and that really did help slow things down – I still had periods, but they were manageable. The word perimenopause wasn't mentioned – my doctor just said that **heavy periods are common in women of my age**. I was just happy that all was well again so didn't really delve any deeper.

I was about 47 when I had a really scary attack of heart palpitations while on a short break with my girlfriends. I had been fast asleep and was awoken by what felt like a train rushing through the room! I immediately leapt up in the bed and looked around wondering where the noise/thumping was coming from – and realised it was coming from inside of me! I tried to take deep breaths and calm myself down and even though my heart wouldn't stop racing, I stayed as calm as I could. Luckily, my friend I was sharing a room with used to be a nurse so she took my pulse and told me not to panic, but that we should get to the hospital as soon as possible. I had a barrage of tests and finally, my heart did stop racing, but it was a really scary episode. When I returned to London, I visited the GP and had some more tests and they all confirmed my heart was strong and healthy and just put it down to 'one of those things.' I then began to do my own research and found out that palpitations could be due to hormone fluctuations. That and the heavy bleeding made me realise I was probably perimenopausal, so I started looking into it more. Funny how you always think 'oh that'll never happen to me"…Oh blimey, how wrong could I have been!

It was when I was 50, along with worsening hot flushes, that the anxiety attacks began and I really freaked out. I had never had anything like it before. I would wake up at 3am with an impending sense of doom and panic with the most awful thoughts going around my head. I would worry that bad things were going to happen all the time and would go dizzy and sweaty when I was driving, imagining that I was going to crash or the bridge I was driving across was going to collapse. I knew that I had to 'get a grip' or get help. The doctor listened and immediately sent me for blood tests to rule out any other problems such as irregularities with the thyroid. When the tests came back, she said that my oestrogen levels were very low –

almost nonexistent – and offered me HRT. We went through my medical records and discussed the pros and cons, and I decided to give them a go.

I've been on **HRT** on and off for 3 years and feel mostly great. I'm not sure whether it's just down to that, but I definitely know my meditation, breathing and workouts are also helping me to keep happy and healthy. If I don't look after myself with a good diet (including treats like wine and cake now and then!), working out and relaxation, it really has a negative impact on my wellbeing. ■

Millicent's Story

'My menopausal journey really started after an operation. I had fibroids. My symptoms started showing in my early forties. I went to a female doctor and asked her to check me out. She did an internal scan and told me she couldn't find anything, and to come back in six months. I went to the doctor again and she scheduled me in for an x-ray, where we found the fibroids. It got to a point where the doctor said these are your options – you can stay like this, *or* you can have a hysterectomy.. It was a difficult decision for me. I felt like parts that made me a woman were being taken out, and I was struggling with the idea of losing them. It's a crazy thought, because obviously I'm still a woman. I had three months to recover, to get my self-esteem and self-worth back.'

'Perimenopause, menopause, whatever you want to call it – I'm there. So, I just decided I accept my fate, I accept I'm going through this. That's part of the battle, I think. If you just roll with it, things become a bit more bearable! I've changed my diet, I'm toning up – I exercise. My daughter during lockdown dragged me into exercising more. She really helps me. Sometimes we do yoga, cardio, stretch exercises. I need to do it because it helps my blood pressure, but it's easier with another person, stops you getting lazy. It helps my health and mental state more than anything, and my physique. I felt really good because it helped me mentally but also boosted my confidence as a woman.'

'I was not always a musician. Music was always a side hobby thing. When I was younger, I saw a lot of women when they got to a particular age who seem to resign themselves to focusing on the family, letting their appearance go. As I approached 40, I had the same experience they had – 'I'm nearly 40, I'm done for, doesn't matter what I wear, I just always feel awful'. Then at some point I decided I'm going to fight against that feeling. On my 40th birthday I went to see my friend playing at the Birmingham Jazz festival. I'm watching him and thinking that we were both in the same jazz band, when I was in my early twenties. He went on to a full-time music career. I didn't see many females with music careers. It took me until I was 42 to decide *I'm going to push this*. I decided to give it five years to see if I can make something with my music. When I made up my mind, things started to happen.. When you are determined, you'll see the doors and you'll do whatever you can do to make it happen.

Don't undervalue your strength, don't doubt yourself, most importantly – *embrace* the new you. Menopause is a new chapter in your life. That's one of the things about the menopause – it's hard, but with the shifts comes more confidence. It makes you more ballsy. You can say what you think. It's a great time to look after yourself. What's going to happen in the body can be hard. There are changes in skin, increased fat deposits, some stuff is going to sag – but if your inner you is happy that sagging is going to look great. Have your nails and hair done if you want to. Doing just that gave me perspective on my body. Understanding what designs work or do not work with your shape and personality has been do helpful when shopping. It's stopped me thinking something is wrong with me. We can't all be Naomi Campbell or Twiggy. We are not them, we are us, and us is beautiful. It's time to reinvent yourself. To be the person you always wanted to be, the you that you put on the back burner. Put yourself central. Don't live in the past, there's no point. It's a new you, and that's wonderful.' ◾

Meg Mathews Stories

1. Titled: The Woman in The Mirror

I don't know who she is, this woman in the mirror. She looks like me but is not the same as me anymore. I know her face, her blue eyes, her skin with maybe few more lines, I see her lips which are still full. Her hair long and blond with just a few grey strands which have been painted over with a great product that makes those grey strands disappear…at least till the next wash. Impossible to run to the hairdresser every 4 weeks. Who can afford such a thing?

Her neck shows some lines- it's lack of hydration. Over fifty-one, got to drink and drink and drink. **Water that is.** It's her eyes which are different.

They don't sparkle anymore. Her heart is beating fast. It's always beating fast now. She has anxieties that overturn her life. It creeps up on her from one minute to the next. As a result, there are days, in which she is scared of leaving the house and it takes real effort in arranging appointments. It's a bit like a full-blown mental health issue, except that it is caused by nothing else but the **drop of estrogen.** A Hormone. A single, simple hormone.

Her mood is like the English weather. Four seasons in one day. It drives everyone around her crazy and challenges loved ones. She can't help it. She really can't. There are badges pregnant woman wear. "baby on board". They are great. When you see a woman with a badge like this in the tube, I get up normally from my seat and make room for her. I remember how tiring it is to be pregnant and how heavy the body feels. It's good to sit down.

I wish there were badges for the pre-menopausal woman too. To alert everyone around of those mood swings. A bit like the owner of dogs who put a sign on their garden door maybe. "Beware of the dog!" My badge would read: "Beware of me, I am pre-menopausal and I don't know the fuck how I'll be reacting to anything you say or do or not do -I might burst into tears, or tear you apart."

At times I feel like I got no layer of skin on my body, nothing to protect my inner self. I am pure and open anything. Pure emotions and soul and feelings. A combination of all of them. I remember my older friend Monica, she used to tell me, that the best time in her life was in her fifties. I get it, kids are grown up, working life in order, time to follow own interests etc. HOWEVER, what she didn't say is, that those nice things will be overshadowed by ANXIETIES. And a sponge brain that doesn't absorb anything at times. Or rather like a sieve that you use to drain spaghetti.

My brain feels like the water that pours out of the tiny holes. Yesterday I asked my doctor to prescribe me a beta-blocker. It slows my fast heartbeat and stops me thinking I might have a heart attack. It helps… It's not a great solution but at least I can carry myself to work without feeling I am going to die any minute. I am considering Hormone Replacement Therapy, but it increases the risk of cancer. *Can't win, can I?*

I can't cope that well with stress anymore either. And it's not the massive stress I used to handle before. You know, the time when you have small children and you have to handle not just yourself but also your children and their appointments and school life and being a great mum and a great wife and go to work and clean the house and do every ones laundry and be interesting by going to interesting places and have interesting friends and do sports and have great hair and write all those Christmas cards to people you don't care about.

No, I don't have any of that any more. Having grown up kids and no husband and no house to clean other than a flat has reduced my stress from 100% to 15%. I also only write 7 Christmas cards. However, at times I can't cope with the minimum of impact life throws at me. I keep looking at the woman in the mirror and I smile. "You know it is not that I don't like you, it's just I wish you would stop worrying about all those things." She smiles back at me.

I feel compassion for her and I am also proud of her, for all those things she managed the last 50 years. "Look, it's ok you feel like a freak at times. Maybe menopause just lets you finally be you. Allows you to be angry now for the things you didn't allow yourself to be angry about before."

I can feel the woman in the mirror is easing up. I can almost see a little sparkle in her eyes. "Thank you, look, I just need more peace. I worked hard on many things over the years, because of this I am a bit tired now. I just want you to allow me to be slower and deal with less. Let me be free to follow my aspirations which I forgot about. Please forgive me for making life an emotional rollercoaster. I promise that it won't last forever."

My heart is beating normal now, and I suddenly feel real and alive as I have never felt before. I feel like I am standing on top of a mountain looking at the most beautiful scenery… *My life. Ahead of me*. Full of me with all the freaking emotions. But real with real values and a sense that I have never been so close to myself before as now. ■

2. Titled: Coming Out about the Menopause

Have I ever told you why I decided to *'come out'* about my menopause? It sounds weird to say it, but it's true, isn't it! You have to at some point tell people, *"I AM MENOPAUSAL"* and it can quite nerve-wracking especially since when I did it I didn't even know how to react to it, let alone how others will.

When I came out about it, everything happened so organically, but I felt like I **had** to talk about it. If you don't do it, if you keep everything for yourself, it could lead to unhealthy habits. Over-eating, unnecessary shopping, or whatever your guilty comfort habit is.

At the time, I worked in interior design, but my mental health was impacting my job. Work, deadlines, emotions... something I could handle so well before, became sometimes too overwhelming. I later realized this was due to the menopause.

So, as I was waking up in the morning I'd ask myself: Do you feel up to talking about how you're feeling about the menopause today? If I answered YES, then I would do it. I was calling people I knew, people around me, and I was talking about my feelings. Most of the time, I was a bit wow, how can I be the only one experiencing this? And this is when you start feeling alone. Not sure if you can even talk because who can relate??

I had mostly mental related **symptoms,** and I was talking about them. When I found out that what I was feeling was all menopause-related, I hadn't been out of the house for 3 months. Inside. Alone. I was just isolating myself, I couldn't face anybody or anything. It was horrendous how I was feeling, and all the emotion I was experiencing. I can't even explain it and wouldn't wish it on my worst enemy, no I DIDN'T want it to happen to anyone. I didn't want anyone else to experience anything similar, my daughter, or another female, feeling invisible.

Then, after 3 whole months, I realized I wanted to do something about it. Not just to help me, but to help if possible every single woman out there who is going through this, or that will at some point go through it. Since I was always an open person, quite comfortable talking in public and about mostly anything, maybe people would start to relate. After all, this is what I was missing, no one was talking about it, and I couldn't be alone feeling this way. I don't think I was being brave, I think this is something I was destined to do.

I realized I had 27 of the 34 symptoms and I thought it could have been a good idea to talk about it. Some of them I never even associated with menopause. The burning mouth sensation I thought was related to the fact that I talk so much. I thought the weight gain was due to my stopping going to the gym. My hair, I thought I need more expensive shampoo. It was not very nice to myself, I found out I gave myself a hard time. My skin was itchy and dehydrated. I thought it was part of getting old, I was struggling with life, I was not able to pack a piece of luggage, pack a bag, anything.

Everything became overwhelming and became essentially bigger than it was. I didn't even want to walk my dogs. Everything became really hard. All I wanted to do was stay in my pajamas. Even opening a letter became difficult. Everything was fearful in my life, it was a very hard time.

I was 49 when I discovered I put it down to stress, but it all started at 42. I don't think I was being brave, I think this is something I was destined to do. As I am a huge advocate for animals, I always thought my life's mission was to help animals. But then I realized God had another job for me, and here I am. For women. And I am only at the beginning of the journey. It took me 2 years to become a strong voice and to be heard. Now we have to prove we need to prevent these feelings from happening. We need to allow people to start HRT on time because prevention is very important.

I am hoping that in the future, everyone will have a letter with menopause info and a *DEXA scan* done routinely at 50. You will get some of the symptoms or all of them or none. Not all of us will have problems, but many women will have osteoporosis and cardiac-related disease because of the menopause. This what I am working for. A future where you go to the GP and say: *"I think I'm going through the menopause"* and it will be enough to get you started on what you really need, before the worst hits. That is what gave me the strength to come out and start talking. ∎

Hilda's Story

I began the menopause at about 46. (The name comes from the Greek words PAUEIN meaning cessation or stopping and MEN meaning month). The first sign was that my periods went haywire. There was no regularity, and boy were they heavy. At one stage, I didn't have one for about six months and then, just to confuse me, the period goddess threw another one in. But that was it ….a kind of long goodbye. Initially, you kind of miss the monthly menses, but it didn't take me long to start rejoicing. I was ready to start the next phase of my life – The Second Spring as they call it in China. Of course, it wasn't all plain sailing. I did suffer from hot flushes that would creep up on me like a sneaky snake. I learned how to cope and wore looser clothes and brought a second t-shirt to school, just in case. But it was the disturbed sleep and night sweats that really affected me. I ate healthily, avoided spicy foods and exercised, but I obviously needed extra help.

My doctor is an advocate of HRT and encouraged me to take it. But I wanted to try a more natural route and so I started on Phyto Soya capsules recommended by my alternative health practitioner. You see, most Japanese women who eat a diet rich in soya don't suffer from hot flushes. Seemingly there isn't even a name for them in Japanese.

The soya plant is rich in isoflavones – natural phyto oestrogens which are vegetable substances similar to female hormones. I bought the capsules in Boots and I noticed recently that they still sell them (a different box and it now uses the word menopause) and, of course, you can get their three-for-two offer. In about three weeks, I noticed a reduction in symptoms and soon they were gone.

After about a year I decided that I must be through it and stopped taking the tablets but within a few weeks, the dreaded sweats were back. So back on the soya for another year and then I tried giving them up again - successfully this time. My blood tests told me I was post-menopausal and I embraced the new phase! ∎

Anonymous Story

Due to me having had a hysterectomy aged 40, it wasn't obvious when I approached menopause. In fact, I wasn't even sure if it would affect me. I was 49 years old, going through a difficult time and attributed my anxiety, irritability, rollercoaster of emotions, decreased libido, low mood and poor sleep to that.

I went to see my GP, who explained that I would still go through the menopause, because despite my hysterectomy, my ovaries were intact. Following some blood tests, my doctor said that I wasn't even pre-menopausal and prescribed me some meds for anxiety. 10 months later, after no significant improvement, I returned to my GP and had further blood tests. Not only was I menopausal, but my hormones had swung so quickly and significantly, that my thyroid gland had become underactive and I was started on thyroid meds, which I am now likely to be on for life. These helped me a lot, my sleep improved and therefore my mood and energy, but unfortunately, the sweats didn't go away.

I continued like this for a few years, until it became so awful that I went back to my GP. My GP said his wife (who was also the senior nurse practitioner at the surgery), was also going through the same and suggested I make an appointment with her, which I did. The nurse was so very understanding and suggested I try HRT. I had read and heard a lot of negativity about HRT and that it increased your chances of cancer. She explained to me that it can increase the risk of breast cancer for women with a family history hereditary the disease. As this did not apply to me, I felt a bit more reassured. She also told me that she was on HRT and if it hadn't been for that, she doesn't think her marriage would have survived! As you can imagine, I thought 'well if it is good enough for her, then it's good enough for me'. Since starting HRT, I have never looked back!

I am now 54 years old, have been on HRT almost 3 years and am beginning to wonder if it is time to come off them. I am scared of 'rocking the boat' and going back to how I was. I know that the sensible thing for me to do, would be to discuss it with my GP or the nurse. That will be the next chapter in my life. Wish me luck! ■

Anonymous Story

I don't even know when I started feeling 'rubbish'. Many women know roughly when they became menopausal. I didn't have a clue. I was busy running a charity in my first CEO role, raising my children on my own and keeping things ticking along at home. I simply didn't join the dots with regards to the symptoms I was experiencing, and that my early symptoms were possibly hormone related. Maybe because in my head I was far too young to be fast tracking my way towards menopause! I do remember my periods getting less and less, but again that refusal to admit that I was a 'woman of a certain age' kicked in. I didn't know at the time that the perimenopause can begin for most women in their early to mid-forties.

I do remember the tiredness and sleep disruption that knocked me for six. I remember feeling so bone achingly tired that the thought of putting one foot in front of the other, particularly at weekends after a long week at work, would sometimes make me want to cry. However, when I went to bed, I would spend all night tossing and turning (due to the hormonal spikes) and watching the clock tick round. Feeling exhausted was no way to start a busy working day, but that became my norm.

It was only when I began to get tremendous joint pain and low mood that I went to the GP. I'd done my own internet research, which had alarmed me to say the least, but I went armed with the self-diagnosis of peri-menopause. Seeing my Doctor wasn't a game changer sadly, but it was a step in the right direction. The Doctor, a much younger woman, wanted to treat my low mood with a combination of counselling – for which there was a several month waiting list – and anti-depressants. Admitting to the Doctor that I was struggling was a big deal for me. I have always been fiercely independent and hated succumbing to any form of 'illness'. My Mum has lived in a care home for over 10 years with advanced dementia, so I had no point of reference in regards to the menopause, to help me make sense of how I was feeling both physically and mentally.

Instead of leaving with a prescription for anti-depressants, I went home, washed my face, changed into my sport kits and joined a 'return to hockey' team. To this day I firmly believe that the combination of physical exercise and a new social group of friends to train and spend time with was my lifeline. Particularly as I now had a genuine reason for those aching joints! I still had bad days. I still had days where new symptoms suddenly cropped up. Chest and leg tremors, dizziness, heart palpitations and tinnitus to name but a few, some scary, some frustrating. I also had to budget for a new wardrobe as my menopausal weight gain took hold, and having prided myself on keeping fit and well, it was difficult when I was unable to control my weight gain.

 For me though when perimenopause was at its peak, I think the hardest thing I had to deal with was fear. An irrational fear that would well up inside of me for no apparent reason until I felt physically sick. Fear that something bad was going to happen to my children was a recurrent theme for me. I remember my son travelling to San Francisco. I checked his flight tracker obsessively until he landed. Panicking in case the flight tracker suddenly disappeared off the screen. I had to stop watching the news as it caused me to worry about the world my children were growing up in. I know as a parent that we worry about our children, but the peri-menopause took this to a whole other level. Uncontrollable, irrational and all-consuming for what felt like the longest time.

I am significantly better now than I was, but do wonder how much longer this will go on for? Who knows, it is different for every woman. What I do know is that the menopause is not an underground movement. It is not a taboo, off limits subject. Nor is it something to make fun of. Particularly when so many women give up work as they can't control their symptoms. Some women give up on life all together.

So that's where we come in, this is my call to action. We are an army of women that can take ownership of this, in whatever small way we are able to. The same as we prepare our children for puberty and our bodies for pregnancy, we need to get our daughters, sisters, nieces and friends ready for this part of a woman's life. Continuing as we are, ignoring symptoms and muddling through is no longer an option. So with that I ask you to talk about, shout about and raise hell fire about this and leave a strong (normalised) legacy for future generations. So here's to strong women. May be know them, may we be them, may we raise them. ∎

Anonymous Story

Throughout my early 40s I just felt 'off'. I didn't feel like myself. When I described the symptoms to my doctor what stood out were my mood swings, hot flushes and feeling bloated. Also my periods were so heavy and painful it was like I was haemorrhaging, which led me to becoming anaemic and very tired. It never occurred to me my problem could be perimenopause – declining levels of the hormone oestrogen in the lead up to menopause. I thought I was too young.

My doctor didn't realise either as he diagnosed a different hormonal problem called polycystic ovarian syndrome – even though I didn't have the other typical symptoms, such as excessive facial hair and obesity. By 45, I was desperate. My gynaecologist said I had no choice but to have my uterus removed. I was about to have a partial hysterectomy and I didn't question it. It was just unbearable and all I wanted was relief. But when I came to in the hospital I suddenly thought, "What have I done?" I realised I would never be able to have another child, and I felt I needed support and counselling but none had been offered.

After the operation, I felt redundant, like an old shoe that was being thrown out. I had lost my identity. I didn't feel like a woman anymore. I felt my husband would no longer find me desirable, even though he had never indicated in any way that he thought that. I had to deal with that on my own, and with the support of my husband. I even asked for support from the church, but they didn't know what to do. Then depression set in. I went to a GP and told him I would cry at the drop of a hat and that I felt strange after the hysterectomy. He said that was normal and put me on a low dose of an antidepressant for six months.

Two years later, aged 47, I was still very unwell. I was working and finishing my Executive Masters of Business Administration (MBA). Critical thinking was very difficult and I found it hard to concentrate. I would also wake in the night and not be able to get back to sleep. I had a mental fogginess and felt I was going crazy. I was angry and upset the whole time. I wondered if it was stress. For a long time I shied away from large assignments at work, and I was basically working part-time because I felt so unwell. I often had to ask for special consideration in the MBA.

So I went to a new doctor, a female GP, who sent me to have a full blood test. When the results came back even she was shocked. She said I'd obviously been battling severe menopause symptoms for a long time because the amount of oestrogen I was producing was negligible. That afternoon, I went home and burst into tears. All of a sudden those feelings of loss, and feeling less of a woman, came back. I was struggling in a lot of ways, even in my interactions with people. Here I was going through a normal stage in a woman's life and I was clueless, and I considered myself to be highly educated. I researched menopause and its emotional effects, but could find nothing at the time. My gynaecologist wanted to prescribe hormone replacement therapy (HRT) in the tablet form. But because I had studied pharmaceutical sciences at university I wanted to do my own research on the different forms of HRT medication.

I am sensitive to the pill and react badly to patches, so I asked for a gel which is applied to the skin on the stomach and upper thighs. I also got a vaginal pessary for associated dryness. From the moment I started using the HRT, I felt better. My energy levels increased, my mood improved, and the fogginess in my mind was gone. I felt normal again. I felt I was back on top of my game. I had more control and it was a huge relief. The HRT gave me enough energy to start exercising again, and I would even go dancing with my girlfriends. Before long I put together a group of friends of different ages as a support group to help us all get through our own challenges with menopause. It felt wonderful to have contributed to diminishing that sense of helplessness and hopelessness. After that it just became a normal but manageable sadness around saying goodbye to my womanhood.

Three years later and I am still on the antidepressant medication, but I have taken other steps to beat the depression for good. A year ago I started practising mindfulness, which is about identifying emotions and accepting them and then letting them go. It is also about being in the moment, no matter what you are doing.

All this lead me to focus on human behaviour and, as part of my MBA, I became an expert in change management, which led me to executive coaching and adopting mindfulness into my professional practice. It's serendipity. I have come from a hard-core senior executive background in the pharmaceutical industry to helping people find their way and become more effective in their careers. It is a big change and it's amazing that menopause had something to do with it. I'm almost 50, I've had a partial hysterectomy, I'm on HRT and I'm very well informed thanks to resources such as the Jean Hailes Foundation. I've made significant changes to my lifestyle in order to manage my symptoms and the sadness. Unfortunately, many of my female friends, colleagues and relatives struggle to find the right information and many find themselves confused and feeling anxious. This is an issue I feel needs more attention, so every woman can feel she is informed and empowered at this time of life.

Dr. Nancy Riley's Story

If you want a scientific article telling you all the physiological details of menopause, keep looking. I am not going to bore you with science. Instead I am going to tell you my story that is also the story of many women as they go through menopause. First, of all the term MENOPAUSE means the 13th month after you stop ovulating and having monthly periods. We have heard our periods called the curse, the visitor, being on the rag and numerous other even less positive things. Most of us never really made friends with our menses or periods. It was just a sign we were not pregnant, and we had to make sure we did not embarrass ourselves with light clothing, or by not having the right sanitary pads or tampons when she decided to roll in.

In my late 30's and early 40's I began to have hot flashes and sudden mood swings. Those sudden mood swings turned me into someone no one really wanted to be around. I found myself consuming large amounts of chocolate, developed broken sleep habits and would lie there night after night listening to my husband snore. I began to take estrogen replacements, black cohosh and evening primrose herbs, and whatever promised to reduce my Godzilletta behavioral habits. Larry, my hubby, ran to the hills when "she" came and he knew instinctively when it was not a good time to have an intelligent conversation. This was called "perimenopausal symptoms."

At the end of my 40's the hot flashes stopped and I thought God had granted me a reprieve from all my past perimenopausal trauma. I had many quiet years with the exception of sleep difficulties due to my changing chemistry. I did not have the mood swings and thought I was ok. Boy, I was really wrong.

I entered my 50s and was told that this was a blissful time for me. I felt I had truly found my voice and was not going to be taken lightly by anyone ever again. I felt I had found my life purpose and passion along with my blooming waist and hips. I knew I would have to do more to stop the fat deposits that often accompany estrogen loss. I began working out more and had a personal trainer to help me build muscle.

I really thought I was FINE. But then I suddenly developed hot flashes again and my urge for sex increased and I was becoming a big bully again. Larry knew once again the other Nancy had come back. I felt at times I was losing my mind. I forgot things, I flew into rages when silly stuff happened. I lost things and became confused and *really* wanted to JUST RUN AWAY. During that time from 50 till around 54, each month around my period I planned my escape, and where I would go when I ran away. In fact I did run off a few times only to find the next day I felt even dumber and more embarrassed to return home and try to explain my odd desires and behavior. Larry learned to just brush it off and when my tears flowed he would comfort me. I really thought I was going to go crazy and had to find a way to get out of my own skin.

Nature and God only gives you so much to endure. I found that after a visit to my physician I had stopped ovulating and periods were about to stop....they did stop for a few months, but then they would come back....however, I did not feel as strange or crazy as I had in past months. At last, I began to feel normal again — whatever that was.

Does this sound familiar to anyone? I have since had conversations with many women who report similar experiences. One woman reported having what she called an out-of-body experience. She thought she was dying and going crazy at the same time. Why women have to go through this is anyone's guess.

I just want to tell you it will pass and you will feel normal again or least feel more comfortable in your skin and where you are. Be sure to talk to other women about what you are experiencing. You will find such valuable support and understanding. It is real and you will come out on the other side feeling wonderful and even more powerful than before. I have been there and won and you will too. **I am OK now and you will be fine too!** ■

Mary's Story

I am a 59 year old Real Estate Agent with somewhat high stress levels. I am single, mom of 3 with 3 grandchildren and one more on the way. I have elderly parents (90 and 84) who also take up some of my time. I walk about 3 to 4 times a week (10,000 KM more or less with hills). I have been in menopause for 2 years now (last period was August of 2019). I can say that I am probably one of the lucky ones except for these few things:

1) I get hot flashes off and on, but they are manageable for the most part. No one can explain or describe to you how those feel. It feels like you are on fire from the inside, I don't love that. They seem to have calmed down though so it doesn't happen too much anymore.

2) My skin, I have rosacea and some eczema on my cheeks. Of course, the lines are more prevalent because my skin is dryer. I can't use most store-bought products on my face, they all seem to give me an allergic reaction.

3) Weight….I put on weight around the middle and a bit here and

there. I eat less and weigh more.

4) Anxiety….I find myself feeling anxious which is new to me and I think this symptom is the worst of them all. It used to be that before a hot flash would come the anxious feeling would alert me it was coming. Now it just comes and goes, and I really can't describe that feeling. I find I get low sometimes for no apparent reason and worry about things more than I used to. Sometimes I wake up and feel so low and anxious that I want to crawl out of my skin. It doesn't last for too long thankfully.

5) Sex drive, what's that??? I really have no desire and if I do have sex the pain is not worth it. It feels like you are being ripped apart. My doctor said to use lubricants but really that doesn't help much. Therefore, my sex life is pretty much dead. I miss even having a desire.

6) Oh, I am also taking a low dose of progesterone and have been through most of this.

I am thankful that my friends and family all get where I am at with this whole thing and therefore cut me some slack. I would say that my mood swings are not too bad.

The only thing I ever heard about menopause was that your period will stop, you might get hot flashes and night sweats (which I don't have) and gain some weight. Everything else has been a big nasty surprise. My older sister who eats mostly vegetables and fish and no sugar has not had any of the things I describe above and therefore it leads me to believe that diet may play a big role in your symptoms. ■

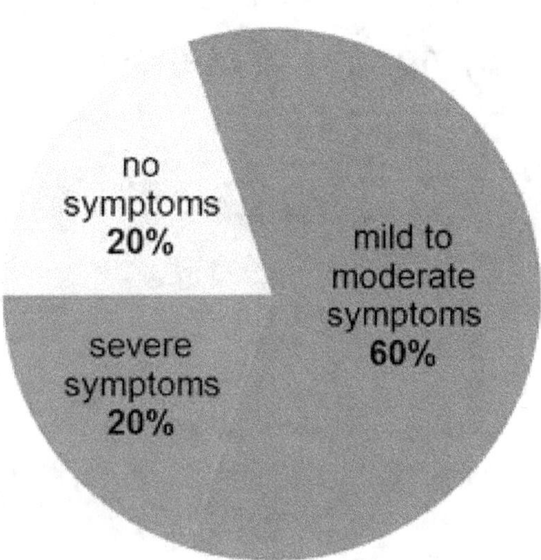

no
symptoms
20%
mild to
moderate
symptoms
60%
severe
symptoms
20%

The 34 Symptoms of Menopause

Common symptoms to expect during menopause.

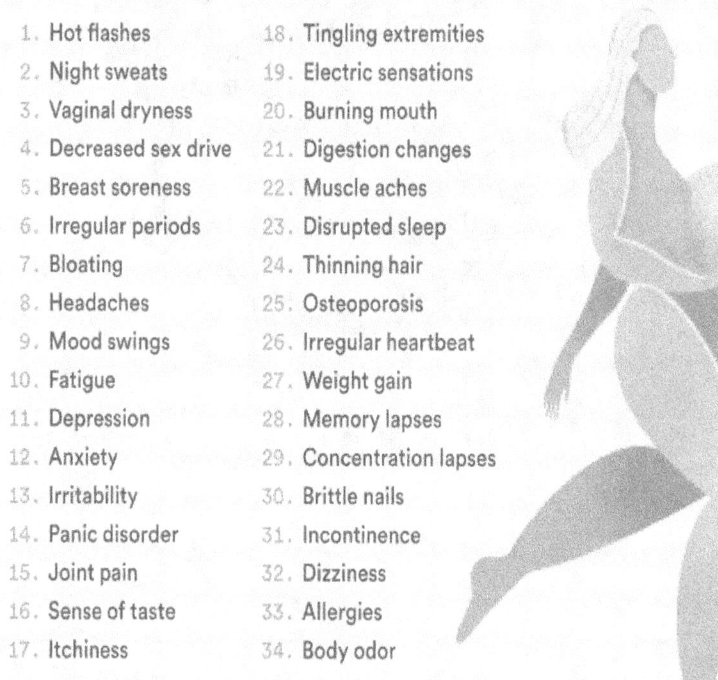

1. Hot flashes
2. Night sweats
3. Vaginal dryness
4. Decreased sex drive
5. Breast soreness
6. Irregular periods
7. Bloating
8. Headaches
9. Mood swings
10. Fatigue
11. Depression
12. Anxiety
13. Irritability
14. Panic disorder
15. Joint pain
16. Sense of taste
17. Itchiness
18. Tingling extremities
19. Electric sensations
20. Burning mouth
21. Digestion changes
22. Muscle aches
23. Disrupted sleep
24. Thinning hair
25. Osteoporosis
26. Irregular heartbeat
27. Weight gain
28. Memory lapses
29. Concentration lapses
30. Brittle nails
31. Incontinence
32. Dizziness
33. Allergies
34. Body odor

PART 5
10 QUESTIONS ANSWERED

Aisling answers 10 questions about Menopause

I'm a mother of 4, I'm 56 and I live in Dublin in a busy household of
a husband and 4 daughters and 1 dog. I run this website My Second Spring
started in 2013 and also **The Silk Pillowcase Company** which I started in
2019. Symptoms can feel like an ambush

1. Your menopause moment? I first noticed hormone action when I was
about 47 - my cycle changed (got longer) and I had some sharp bursts of
irritability, breast tenderness, fuzzy head/brain fog - symptoms that
reminded me initially of pregnancy.

2. Secret menopause or open book? I was the first in my group to
mention menopause and at first, I was very reticent, embarrassed and shy
about talking about it. People's reactions were interesting and most people a
bit shocked that I was talking about it. It's still not a comfortable topic.
Some women see it as weakness to have symptoms or 'give in' to
menopause. Although this has changed a lot since 2013.

3. Your symptoms? My symptoms lasted about 6 years later they are very
variable - some days lack of confidence, other days irritability, the odd night
sweat. They can feel like an ambush. They have never been too intense. I
eventually hit full menopause at 53.

4. Your approach? My approach is to work on myself and try to improve
my diet (less sugar, less coffee and less wine, more vegetable and
fish protein, more vegetables); stay fit and move every day - I try to move
as much as possible and include stretching and strengthening exercises in
my regime as well as cycling and swimming and reduce stress where
possible. I take supplements for overall health and hormone balance in

particular. My GP suggested that I was a candidate for HRT because my FSH level is 49 but as my symptoms are not very limiting I didn't consider this option at that time. I've never liked taking artificial hormones. The pill made me moody and I put on weight. There are now far more options in terms of gels, patches and pessaries that I would consider if my symptoms were limiting my everyday life. I have used homeopathy to manage symptoms.

The good, the bad, the ugly

5. The pros? Menopause has given me an opportunity to look at my life and the way I'm living and to shift some aspects. My symptoms have been guides. For example I know that some of my irritability was around being a full-time mother led me to set up My Second Spring. Night sweats come on when I have wine in the evening so I've cut back. I wake at night when I've had too much coffee too late at night. I love to eat so I need to keep moving to keep weight gain at bay.

6. The cons? Feeling fuzzy-headed/brain foggish forgetting things and feeling low in confidence can be very destabilizing. At times I was convinced I was getting Alzheimer's/dementia even though I rationally knew that the brain symptoms were hormone-related. I didn't always feel or think rationally!

7. What's helped? Taking supplements have helped my tiredness and given me more energy - I discovered through a blood test that I was v deficient in B12. Exercise has been brilliant in feeling empowered and strong and also the daily high that it brings which helps reduce stress. In some ways I feel more body fit and confident that any other time in my life. I was never a sporty person and lacked confidence in that area.

8. What hasn't? My doctor suggesting that I was a candidate for HRT even though I was managing symptoms and had told her I didn't want to take it at that time. I felt annoyed by that as she clearly wasn't listening to me. I since moved doctors and have found a like-minded GP. I think menopause is a time to make sure you have confidence in your medical support for the future.

9. Best menopause advice? My guiding light was Dr Christiane Northrup

The Wisdom of Menopause as it gave me a wide, balanced and positive outlook on menopause.

10. Sum up menopause in three words: Massive personal development - aka My Second Spring. ■

Loretta Dignam answers 10 questions about menopause

I'm 56, and a divorced mother of two children. I raised my son, 25, and daughter, 17, on my own for 15 years - with the help of course of some great childminders and au pairs, as I worked full-time outside the home. We have Bichon Frise dogs, Bounty and Twix (named from my time with Mars, the chocolate business).

I have worked most of my career at Marketing Director level in blue-chip multinationals: Mars Inc, Diageo, Kerry Group and Jacob Fruitfield, and won Marketer of the Year in 2011 for my work on turning around the Jacob's biscuit brand. I've lectured in the Michael Smurfit Business school on their Executive MBA programme; joined the board of The Abbey theatre in 2015, chaired its Gender Equality Committee. Last year, I set up The Menopause Hub in Dublin.

I am passionate about sports, I've coached basketball for several years and I love skiing - I go with my daughter and friends to France every year. Last year my daughter and I completed a 250km charity cycle in Vietnam for Plan International - incredible! And I've really enjoyed getting into dancing via local charity Strictly Come Dancing events.

1. Your Menopause Moment? The month before I turned 50, my periods stopped…forever. I never had another period after that. And since I had never even heard of the perimenopause, I have no idea what symptoms I had leading up to that. Then one month after my periods stopped, the hot flushes began. Relentless. 20 – 30 a day plus, at night. The duvet was on, then it was off, on, off, all night long. The hot flushes were the only symptoms I associated with the menopause at the time, it took me a while to connect my other symptoms.

2. Secret menopause or open book? At the time I didn't want anyone to know that I was menopausal, for two reasons. Firstly, I didn't want people to know my age, and secondly, well let's face it …are there any positive associations with being a menopausal woman? I did chat to my close friends, none of whom had experienced any symptoms or if they did, were mild, so they couldn't really empathise.

I turned to Doctor Google and found out about Sage, Black Cohosh and the Ladycare Menopause Magnets in Boots. I also consulted the local health shop and Valerian root was suggested. I tried them all. The Chinese herbalist recommended Dong Quai. I cut down on coffee, tea, alcohol. Increased my exercise, slept in a cool room….need I go on? I tried all of the 'alternatives' before I finally, after 3 long years, went to see my GP. Needless to say, now I am an open book! I want to champion the menopause cause and break the last remaining taboo in women's health.

3. Your symptoms? Looking back and knowing what I know now, my symptoms were many and varied:, hot flushes, broken sleep, pains in my ankles, dry skin, thinning eyebrows, getting up in the night to go to the loo, leakage on laughter and sneezing, dry eyes, (prompting 3 trips to the A&E department), unusual blood test results, high cholesterol, low thyroid, fatigue, low energy, receding gums, loss of libido and irritability. And an overall lack of va va voom, vitality, mojo …whatever you might call it.

Luckily for me, I didn't have what many other women experience - anxiety, depression, panic attacks, loss of confidence and mood swings. Interestingly, I was also diagnosed with asthma, which I have read is connected to menopause, but I'm not sure how widely known nor scientifically proven it is. To me, with hindsight, I see the menopause as the breaking down of my body. I had put a lot of it down to age and/or stress. These lost hormones have been described to me as the oil for the engine. None of us would consider driving our car without oil, would we?

4. Your approach? After 3 years of symptoms, which I can only describe as relentless and exhausting, I felt like I had experienced a slow puncture. Life was ebbing out of me. Eventually, I went to my regular Doctor and began the process of discovering HRT (Hormone Replacement Therapy).

I had a false start with the first HRT solution I tried, a combined HRT patch, which was not effective. I discovered through research that I am progesterone sensitive, which explained why I could never take the pill. Every time I tried, I felt so bad in oh so many ways, and had to come off it. How I only have two children is a miracle!! I also tried the Mirena Coil, which was a disaster for me, when I broke out in volcanic spots, I decided it had to go. It only lasted for 5 weeks.

I then went to see a doctor who specialised in menopause and tried separate body identical hormones, initially oestrogen and progesterone. After a couple of months, testosterone was added into the mix. After about 6 months, during which the dosage was tweaked, usually increased, I was feeling back to my old self, all of the symptoms were gone. It was a fantastic feeling.

I turned to HRT as a last resort as I had previously believed it was risky and ineffective. In the quest for something that would alleviate my symptoms and improve my quality of life, I read everything I could get my hands on about HRT, the pros and cons, and the myths, too. The truth, as I see it, is that the benefits of HRT far outweigh the risks for most women. My symptoms were sorted out but I have also protected my long term bone health, cardiovascular health and cognitive health in the process. That should mean reduced risk for osteoporosis, heart attack and Alzheimer's.

5. The pros? Bio identical HRT worked for me. My troublesome menopause symptoms were all reversed. And the longer term benefits - my bone, heart and cognitive health are all protected. I am confident in my choice. It works for me.

6. The cons? In 2002, results from the now-famous Women's Health Initiative, a long term US women's health study, pointed to a small increased risk of developing breast cancer associated with the use of HRT.

More recent and specific research has now suggested that in fact, the risk is extremely low. When I dig deep into all the available research today, I find have a greater risk of getting breast cancer if I drink two units or more of alcohol a day, or if I am overweight or obese, than if I am on HRT. So each woman must weigh the benefits and risks for herself before deciding on a treatment option. I'd say - do your research and look for recent clinical studies.

7. What helped? HRT helped with my symptoms. And I wish I had known about how effective it is 3 years ago, I would have started while I was still peri-menopausal. Effectively, I believe I wasted 3 years of my health life.

8. What didn't?   Not speaking openly about menopause, not seeking help earlier. What definitely didn't help me was natural, alternative solutions or lifestyle changes. That's just my experience. That's why I set up The Menopause Hub, to do the 'leg-work' for other women, to short-cut it all.

9. Best menopause advice? Two 'aha' moments for me were when I saw the list of symptoms of the menopause all together. Up until that, I had not connected the dots. As a result, I created a Symptom Checker. It is astonishing when you read the full list of circa 40 symptoms; physical, emotional, psychological and sexual.

The second was when I saw the British Menopause Society's Women' Health Concern chart – Understanding the Risk of Breast Cancer. (See below) It put HRT in context and very much put my mind at ease. We have both of these on display at The Menopause Hub and share them with the women who visit us.

10. Sum up the menopause in three words: Loss of vitality! ■

Ravi answers 10 questions about Menopause

1. Your menopause moment? I am still not officially IN menopause, but perimenopause started around age 42 with hot flashes. I am now 51, periods still erratic, but feel like I'm over the worst of it... fingers crossed.

2.Secret menopause or open book? I am definitely not a "suffer in silence" type...lol. After I figured out what was going on, and how earth-shattering my symptoms were becoming, I spoke out candidly, and regularly to my husband and son, to my girlfriends, posted on social media (crickets chirping) and was SHOCKED at how most of my girlfriends were not experiencing their symptoms yet or were too embarrassed to talk about it!! I often felt very alone. My husband and son were wonderful, and my close girlfriends were good listeners, but very few admitted to having as hard a time with it as I was having...

3. Your symptoms? I now understand that every woman's perimenopausal symptoms are different. For me, I could handle the PHYSICAL symptoms (hot flashes, heavy bleeding, heart palpitations, etc), but what was the hardest for me were the EMOTIONAL and COGNITIVE symptoms (high anxiety, brain fog, fatigue)... it became so difficult that I had to make some drastic changes in my work and am now working on a career change that does not involve so much multi-tasking and stress.

4. Your approach? When my PCP/GP was not helpful (she is a woman and I love working with her but she was not helpful with this...), I ended up seeing a naturopath who put me on a load of supplements, bioidentical hormones and diagnosed me with severe anemia so added iron supplements. It made a HUGE difference! But it was very expensive as much of it wasn't covered by my health insurance. And the more research I did on HRT/bioidentical hormones the more I understood that it's really messing with "Mother Nature" and they really don't know what the long term effects are. Based on my personal beliefs of trying to stay as "natural" as possible, I used the hormones/supplements to get me over the worst symptoms and then stopped taking them. I no longer need to take them because I've made some major lifestyle changes that are working WITH this new normal instead of being stubborn and trying to "push that boulder up a hill"?

5.The Pros? Helped decrease my anxiety and gave me more energy/decreased fatigue/brain fog.

6. The Cons? Expensive and unknown long-term effects (cancer?)

7. What's helped? Hormones, iron and other supplements given by naturopath, accepting the new normal and making lifestyle changes (including decreasing stress, changing careers, focusing on creativity - writing, painting, etc, focusing on how to "give back" by sharing the knowledge I have acquired through the years both professionally and personally).

8. What hasn't? Taking tons of supplements/HRT long term, being stubborn and refusing to change/accept/move on.

9. Best menopause advice?
See perimenopause as a time of growth, asking you to change and fully grow into the Wise Woman you are becoming. Do not fight this change, accept that it will be painful at times, but it is guiding you towards a new life and higher self.

10. Sum up Menopause in 3 words:
Difficult, lonely, transforming. ■

Andrea McLean answers 10 questions about menopause

1. Your menopause moment? My first symptoms of perimenopause started when I was about 37/38. My Mum started at 40 so I was prepared for that.

2. Secret Menopause or open book? I'm quite a keep-it-to-myself person so I was quiet about it at that time. But then a few years later when I had my hysterectomy, my colleague encouraged me to announce that on air on Loose Women - and we had an unprecedented response - that lead to me becoming something of a poster girl for menopause! I wrote my book Confessions of a Menopausal Woman as a result. But even now I don't necessarily talk about it unless someone wants me to.

3. Your symptoms? Night sweats were the absolute worst, then carrying on into the day. Then the next worst was mood swings - I'm normally quite steady but I became irritable over the smallest thing and rage like nobody's business. I still have that now - in fact, I had that experience earlier today with a taxi driver who wouldn't put on the air conditioning and I was getting hotter and hotter!

4. Your approach? Mix and match, a little bit of this a little bit of that. Definitely look at your diet. Try and cut out as much sugar as you can – never mind being fat or anything like that it's to do with spikes in energy levels, hormone levels. I know this sounds really dull but try to be moderate in all things so a bit of caffeine, a bit of alcohol, a bit of cheese. Don't cut anything out because you'll just crave it. Try to bring things down to a sensible level. And the same with exercise – just keep flipping along don't take on a big mad plan. I read a really good thing recently: rather than saying I should have done this I should have done that, make a promise to yourself and say to yourself I promise I'm going to do this and make it tiny, tiny, tiny so that you keep it. Having read that I made a promise to myself, and a promise is a promise, so now I have to keep it.
I've bought myself one of these resistance bands and I have it rolled up beside my toothbrush and my promise is that I do 30 squats every morning

when I'm brushing my teeth. Sometimes I see the band there beside my toothbrush and I'm not in the mood but I go 'but I promised!', so I have to do it. But if I said 'Oh I should have done that' then I feel bad but I can't break a promise so I just do it and I never regret it. I only ever regret not doing it.

5. The pros? The big pro is acceptance - because you realise you have to kind of surrender. We fight so often throughout every other part of our lives. Then you get to a point when you realise, I am going through menopause and I have to do something about it. You can't just keep pushing against it. And then it's actually an opportunity to look at every other part of your life. Whether it's your food, your exercise, your relationships… everything.

6. The cons? Every other part of it!!

7. What's helped? For me, I had to really make an effort to keep on top of the mental side of things. I've been affected more mentally than physically. It has made me tune in to myself a lot more. Rather than just keeping going, keeping going, like I was. I now have to acknowledge that I'm going to fall down, I'm going to tip over. When that happens I go to a very dark, very anxious place. So it's now realising that before it happens and keeping on top of everything.

8. What hasn't? Not keeping on top of things. Ignoring little flags along the way.

9. Best menopause advice? Know the symptoms - there are 34 of them! And realise that you're not going mad, that these odd symptoms could be the menopause and then - 'Great!' because you know it will pass.

10. Sum up menopause in three words!
Time for change! ■

PART 6
LINGER LONGER STORIES

Enjoy these deep dives into personal experience…..

No One Told Me Exactly What to Expect From Menopause. But the Messages I Did Get Were Very Wrong

BY <u>DARCEY STEINKE</u>

I was 50 when I woke in my dark attic bedroom in Brooklyn, my heart speeding and my body incandescent with heat. I did not feel simply hot, no, I was being smothered by an internal fire that seemed to pool inside my body like lava. At first I thought it was a heart attack. After more flashes, over my morning bowl of oatmeal, as I rode the subway under the East River and while I taught, I realized it was not a heart attack. It was a hot flash. I had entered menopause, that fraught transition in every woman's life, known in an earlier time as The Dangerous Age.

The heat was uncomfortable, but the aura of anxiety just before each flash was worse. I felt as if a shard of a different reality had been thrust into my current one. I also had insomnia: I had trouble both getting to sleep and staying asleep. There were sexual changes as well. Positions I once enjoyed were no longer comfortable. And I thought about sex less. The daily tug toward intimacy had vanished.

Earlier life stages, going through puberty and giving birth, had opened up new worlds, the excitement of sexuality and motherhood. But menopause arrived without absorbing directives. Instead of new obsessions and responsibilities, I felt a nothingness. It's a void created in part by our oversexed patriarchal culture, a world that has little respect for older women. Valued most for our sexuality and role as mothers many women feel, once that phase is over, as I did. Marginalized. The message, never stated directly but manifesting in myriad ways, is an overwhelmingly nihilistic one: your usefulness is over. Please step to the sidelines.

As my estrogen lessened, I also felt my femininity fraying. I was called "sir" twice. Once by a parking lot attendant and another time by the boy who bagged my groceries. I don't possess the strong female signifiers I once did. My hair is no longer long and shiny, my skin no longer smooth. I wear more androgynous clothing and rarely put on makeup. I've lost interest in "doing" my female gender, in propping it up. At times I feel another body slipping out from my original one. Once, when coming up from the subway, I saw a reflection of an older man in the bodega window. I stared for a few seconds before I realized it was me.

I searched for books that might help me understand what was happening to me. I read Suzanne Sommers' *The Sexy Years* and Gail Sheedy's *Silent Passages*. Both are fear-based. Both authors are frantic to keep the veneer of a fertile femininity intact. Both books treat menopause like a disease, something to be cured, not a transition to be celebrated. Neither offers a sympathetic understanding of what women are going through physically, emotionally or spiritually. Sommers and Sheedy are so concerned with propping up their femininity with hormones, that they miss the profounder subtleties of the menopausal tradition. I found trans memoirs, by men and women who were transitioning, better at helping me understand my own hormonal transformation. In his book *The Testosterone Files*, Max Wolf Valerio writes about his move from female to male, calling it "a unique intensive fire." As he moves out from under the veil of estrogen he feels "a bright clarity." To Valerio hormonal changes are an "adventure." He even goes so far as to compare his transition from female to male to menopause. "A woman I know going through menopause reports that she too feels this clarity and that sometimes she feels like a wise old owl, who can see for a very long distance."

Valerio helped me see hormonal changes as a gain rather than a loss. But it was an animal, a sea creature, who taught me the most about post-menopausal leadership. Female killer whales, as well as narwhals and short-finned pilot and beluga whales, are the only other animals who go through menopause. Older killer female whales have a sharp menopause and then go on to live another 30 or 40 years. One whale, J2, also known as Granny, lived to be 104. The post-reproductive females lead their pods—complex, cohesive family groups—particularly in times when salmon, their main food source, is scarce. "Elder females," an article in the journal *Nature* read, "hold ecological knowledge and all whales, even younger males, prefer to follow the older females."

J2 and the other post-reproductive pod leaders taught me that it's not menopause itself that is the problem but menopause as it's experienced under patriarchy. On television and in films, hot flashes are a comedic skit akin to a man slipping on a banana peel. In *Mrs. Doubtfire*, Robin Williams' fake breasts catch on fire and, using two pan lids, he eventually puts the fire out. He stands disheveled, his chest smoking. "My first day as a woman," he says, "and I'm already having hot flashes." Women too make fun of menopause. On Etsy you can buy buttons that read "Beware of Temper Tantrums" and "Out of Estrogen: Approach at Your Own Risk." Online jokes abound. "Q: What is ten times worse than a woman in menopause? A: Two women in menopause."

Only recently have female celebrities begun to speak with candor about the change. Gwyneth Paltrow feels that there are not enough menopausal role models, "Menopause gets a bad rap and needs a bit of rebranding." Whoopi Goldberg felt forced to examine the negative people in her life and cut them out. Cynthia Nixon found the change freeing. "There has been no sadness for me, because once you hit 50, you're done." Still men negate and diminish our passage. In 2013 comedian Jeff Allen told jokes about lying next to his menopausal wife in bed and "dreaming about the good old days of PMS." More recently French author Yann Moix said that 50-year-old women were invisible to him, that they were "too old" to love: "The body of a 50-year-old is not extraordinary at all."

Menopause is not a punch line. All women will go through this change, and it's important as a culture that we learn to understand and honor menopause, not make fun of it. It's an isolating period, and lame humor makes it worse. A recent study by Myra Hunter, emeritus professor of clinical health psychology at Kings College London published in the journal Menopause, found that women in the workplace are worried about being made fun of. "There's embarrassment and anxiety," she said, "about being joked about and a big concept is hiding symptoms in fear of being ridiculed." Why should women, in the workplace or at home, who are going through a normal female life stage be teased or demeaned?

Beyond this everyday attitude toward menopause that it is funny or gross, there is also the idea pushed by some drug companies that menopause is not mandatory. Preying on vulnerable women who may feel disoriented by what is happening to their bodies, they argue that the right way to go through the change is not to change at all. They define menopause, a female life cycle no different than puberty or birth, as a disease, a dangerous condition that can only be cured by hormone treatment. There is a difference, though, between female health and what will keep us chemically configured as if still fertile.

I knew very little as I started menopause. When I was a teenager, I saw my mother in her late '40s experience it when she stalked our un-air-conditioned Virginia ranch house wearing only a house dress, her face pink and sweat covered. When asked what was wrong, she'd say nothing. Shame made it impossible for my mother to even say the word menopause, and while now we may be more open about the female body and its transitions, many women still feel silenced and degraded by a culture that sees our changing bodies as useless.

Menopause does not negate, but dilates what it means to be a woman. No longer defined as a sex object, I am now so much more. Menopause is as much a spiritual transition as a physical one — with every flash I am reminded that my life in this body will not go on forever. This has been valuable. I want to be more expansive in the decades I have left. Out from under the haze of female hormones, I am a new creature, one closer to my former fierce little girl self. I feel a return to that essential me I had to leave behind once the huge disruptive force of puberty kicked in. I see now that my breeding years were an aberration rather than the norm. I can no longer reproduce but my body is far from over.∎

Haley Cockman - A teenage menopause story
What it's like to hit menopause at the young age of 14.

14 years old and told I had gone through the menopause… yep that's right 14 years old.

I will never forget that day, sitting on the bed in a hospital room waiting for the consultant to come into me and my Mum saying those words. My Mum bawling her eyes out and me comforting her asking her to not cry as it's ok. Thing is it wasn't ok, but then I had no clue what the Consultant was even talking about.

At the age of 12 I started my periods like a normal teenager. Then after a year they just stopped. I was struggling to concentrate at school and the nights were hell. Waking up dripping with sweat and just feeling weird. That's literally how I described it to my Mum one day. I don't feel like me Mum, I feel weird. So off we went to the Doctor's. I explained what was going on and I was referred for a blood test and an ultrasound. Then two weeks later a consultant gynaecologist confirmed I had gone through my Menopause and that I needed to start taking HRT tablets.

I was told I had a womb but a small one and that they could only find one ovary. That was the first and the last time I was going to see my consultant. I am now 39 years old. I literally have never been contacted since. Not given any follow up appointments, no help, no guidance to understand what had happened to me nothing. Put on Prempak C and left to just get on with it.

Even when Prempak C was discontinued a few years back I wasn't even informed by my Doctor. The pharmacist told me when I went to pick up my meds. Meds, may I add that I have to pay for… which I find astonishing. I need to take these daily and I had none left so luckily after a long phone call I managed to get in with a GP the next day. Who then told me there was no exact alternative and she was putting me on another brand. But that was horrendous. All my levels went crazy and my symptoms returned, and my bleeds were so painful. I then was changed onto Femoston which I now take and luckily have no problems with. Even my bleed isn't as painful anymore as I have to have one monthly to keep the lining of my womb working properly, in-case I was to decide I wanted to try IVF. Something I have decided against, as I cannot go through a grieving process again if it wasn't successful.

As a child I needed to learn what it all meant, and back then there was hardly anything on the internet to read and even to this day limited material to a teenager experiencing this happening to them. This needs addressing as I felt lost for years as I just didn't understand it all. Medical professionals looked at me like I was some sort of freak. If I was given a pound for the amount of times a doctor or nurse has said to me "you poor girl" when I answer the dreaded question… "what medication do you take". I would have had loads of work done on myself. Which leads me on to how I have felt growing up… hating what I saw looking back at me in the mirror. The one job a woman is given to do, and I couldn't even do that properly. I felt like a failure. A failure as a woman.

I can't say I grew up depressed I just learnt how to cope. I grew up not liking my appearance. I suppose I felt insecure about myself. I struggled with relationships with guys as I knew I had it looming over me that one day I was going to have to tell them. Even when I did tell them or my friends neither understood. I even lost a friend over it as she said I was lying and that it was a sick thing to make up! Charming ay… The response I got from the close few I did tell was always the same… It will happen one day mate, loads of women are told they can't have kids and they do.

Nobody understood what I was saying. Because no one was/is educated enough, No one knows what it means. Even to this day people still do not understand. So, in my words I say it how it is…. To produce a baby, you need an egg and a sperm, and I don't have eggs, end of.

Literally one week ago I decided I was ready to talk about my experience out loud and to try and get this recognised more. To get people to speak out and not hide it all inside, because you feel everyone will be gossiping about you.

Unfortunately, it happens to all of us females one day. There is no set age limit on it, which I am living proof of…..

Today, Hayley is over 40 and dedicated to raising awareness around premature menopause. ■

Jeanne Muchnick's Story

Titled: I've gone slightly insane…..

Thanks to menopause, I've gone slightly insane. As in full blown freaking out/screaming/crying/ semi-hysterical over the smallest, most innocuous things.

Case in point: Two weeks ago when my husband ate the sushi I had bought for myself. No, I didn't leave a note on the fridge warning him not to eat it. And no, I never mentioned to him that I had a particular craving for a California roll and under no circumstance was he to touch it. In my crazed state, I just assumed he'd know.

So when I came home after a long, hard day at work and it wasn't there – this after practically ripping the entire refrigerator apart — I went into full-out hysteria mode as in "WHERE IS MY SUSHI????"

And then – with a glare in my eye straight out of a horror movie: "What do you mean you ate it??? I do everything around this house, you couldn't have saved me my one little tray of sushi???? What were you thinking???"

The rant went on: "I was been dreaming…DREAMING of eating that all day. ALL DAY!!! Now what will I have? I specifically bought that earlier to enjoy TONIGHT!"

"What about pasta?" asked my normally sensitive hubby. "Or a Trader Joe's pizza? I can heat the oven up for you."

"How can I eat something with tomato sauce when I was yearning for sushi?" I bellowed. "YEARNING???? I'm not in a tomato mood. I wanted Asian. That's why I bought the sushi and left it there. For me. That was MY order. You never go for California rolls."

"What are you talking about?" he asked. "I eat California rolls."

"Not a lot, you don't," I countered angrily. "Not enough that I'd think to tell you not to eat it."

And then came the sobs. Real crocodile tears, in fact. Kids are going hungry all over the world, people are losing their mortgages left and right and there I was – 50 years old in my nice Dutch Colonial kitchen — literally crying because I couldn't think of anything else I wanted to eat and I was hungry. As in blood sugar falling fast hungry. As in hormonal hell-watch-out-because-the-earth-is-falling hungry.

"You need to go out now," I told him. "NOW! I want the same exact sushi– and I don't care how many stores you have to go to to find it."

"Now?" he asked. He was already in his sweats. "Can I run to Stop & Shop?"

"Are you kidding me? The sushi sucks there," I said. "You'll need to go the Food Emporium where I was or one of the sushi restaurants on Mamaroneck Avenue," I said.

"GO!" I said with a push. "I mean it. NOW." Stiff cold body language. Arms crossed. Insane Asylum glare.

"Jeesh," he said…a bit scared I think. Even my hair was electric – the better to go with my bugged out eyeballs which screamed "HURRY! I'm in menopausal meltdown!!!"

And that's just one example of the nutty menopause moments I've had of late where I swear my body and mind have become inhabited by aliens. Which brings me to this — my invitation to share your craziest, most embarrassing, most hilarious menopause moments.

Whadda ya say ladies? Don't be shy. Are you irritable? Feeling out of sorts? Done anything off the wall? You're not alone. Let's share. Or do you want me to go into my "*Why do you refuse to buy a GPS?*" story where we got major league lost in a bad DC neighborhood? My kids STILL refer to this episode as "Remember The Time Mom Went Insane?" ■

Rebecca Doyle's Story, Age 49

This HR Director at Opera Australia first began experiencing perimenopausal symptoms in March 2020.

"I had gained weight, was having trouble sleeping and suffering with mood swings; someone pushing in a supermarket queue would make me irrationally angry," Doyle recalls.

"I went to see my GP, and they prescribed me HRT. I'm not sure whether it was the timing and stress of that first lockdown or just because the treatment wasn't for me, but it actually made my symptoms worse."

While swimming and intermittent fasting have since helped, it was a beautician enquiring about Rebecca's acne who suggested she try a natural remedy.

"She asked about my pimples and whether I was going through perimenopause. She recommended the Happy Hormones supplement and while not all my symptoms went away, I began sleeping better which has also helped my general anxiety."

Dr Joanna Sharp, a specialist General Practitioner who consults for online menopause clinic My Juniper, says that a change in the condition of your skin, like Rebecca experienced, could be due to hormonal fluctuations associated with menopause.

"When we think of menopause, we often think of the common symptoms such as hot flushes, vaginal dryness, low mood and weight gain, but there are actually quite a few other symptoms to consider," Dr Sharp says.

Dr. Sharp says that while 20 percent of women will sail through menopause, 80 percent will experience symptoms and 25 percent of them will be severe.

She says that these three 'invisible' and unusual symptoms, not commonly associated with perimenopause and menopause, are worth looking out for:

1. Formication.

"The word formication comes from the Latin word 'formica' which means ant. So this is literally the feeling of having ants crawling on or under your skin which is very unpleasant. This is because of the change in your hormones and dry skin and it may cause intense itching and irritation."

2. Brain fog and light-headedness.

"Similar to 'baby brain' or the changes that your brain goes through as a teenager, brain fog is a completely normal part of menopause and the shift in hormones. It is hard to say what causes the light-headedness but again it could be the change in your hormone levels."

3. Joint pain.

"As oestrogen levels drop during menopause, inflammation of the joint can increase and cause pain. Old injuries or diseases may contribute to joint pain, so I would always suggest further investigation to discover the cause."

Dr Sharp says that the key to dealing with perimenopause and menopause is to consider that every woman experiences different symptoms and it's essential to seek professional advice to consider your overall health during midlife.

"It's a very individual journey. I often refer to it as the 'menopuzzle' and so my patients and I work together on their unique treatment plan to bring all the pieces together," Dr Sharp says.

"This might include factoring in lifestyle elements such as adding more calcium to their diet or doing strength and weight based exercise."

Dr Sharp believes that there is still too much fear and shame around midlife and menopause and that it should instead be a time to refocus on what you want from life.

"When we go through puberty, we learn about this phase of life at school. When we have babies, we go to antenatal classes. We need an equivalent for menopause to help ease fear and embrace and celebrate the change."

Rebecca Doyle agrees that we need to be more open about menopause symptoms to help change the narrative and encourage more women to seek help.

"Considering all women have to go through menopause, it seems crazy to me that we don't talk about it more. I think this represents the fact that many female health issues have been neglected for too long.

"There has long been this feeling of embarrassment or shame around menopause, which is ridiculous when you consider what a privilege it is to age.

"We are good at celebrating the teenage years and pregnancy and birth, so why not menopause?" ■

The Secret Power of Menopause by Liza Mundy
Why the end of fertility doesn't mark the start of decline—and may even help explain our success as a species.

DON'T TRY TO TELL THIS to a mother sitting in the bleachers during a four-hour swim meet; or enduring a birthday party involving toddlers and craft projects; or resting in an armchair on a peaceful evening, savoring the heft of a tiny body and the scent of an infant's freshly washed hair. Interminable or sweetly languid though they may feel in the moment, the childbearing years are startlingly brief. Fertility, which typically ends in a woman's mid-40s, occupies less than half of her adult life. And then, if she's lucky, she has 30 or 40 years in which to do something else.

Most people don't realize how unusual humans are, in the way that non-reproductive females (how shall I put this?) persist. Females of most other species can bear young until they die, and many do, or at best enjoy a brief respite from breeding before death. This is true not only of creatures you might expect, such as rabbits, but also of long-lived mammals such as Asian elephants, and of primates such as gorillas and chimps. The odd exceptions—the Japanese aphid, for example, enters a "glue bomb" stage after her reproductive phase, ready to immobilize a colony . The mystery of why women go on and on and on after their procreative function has ceased has occupied some of the great minds of the ages. I am sorry to report that many of those minds have not been forward-thinking. "It is a well-known fact … that after women have lost their genital function their character often undergoes a peculiar alteration" and they become "quarrelsome, vexatious and overbearing," Sigmund Freud pronounced. The male-dominated medical community of the mid-20th century was similarly dismissive. "The unpalatable truth must be faced that all postmenopausal women are castrates," opined the gynecologist Robert Wilson, who elaborated on this theme in his 1966 best seller, *Feminine Forever*. The influential book, it later emerged, was backed by a pharmaceutical company eager to market hormone-replacement therapy.

Even the architects of the sexual revolution were fixated on fertility as a marker of femininity, an attitude that seems doubly unfair coming from the people who gave us the pill. "Once the ovaries stop, the very essence of being a woman stops," wrote the psychiatrist David Reuben in 1969 in *Everything You Always Wanted to Know About Sex but Were Afraid to Ask*, adding that the postmenopausal woman comes "as close as she can to being a man." Or rather, "not really a man but no longer a functional woman."Little wonder that women writers have felt the need to weigh in over the centuries. A few took an upbeat approach. At the age of 41, having just given birth to her sixth child, the suffragist Elizabeth Cady Stanton wrote her friend Susan B. Anthony in 1857 to say that their best activist years lay ahead. "We shall not be in our prime before fifty & after that we shall be good for twenty years at least." Others were less sanguine. At 54, writing her memoir, Simone de Beauvoir gloomily prepared to say "goodbye to all those things I once enjoyed"; women, Freud had taught her, become miserable and sexless as they age. Betty Friedan, Gloria Steinem, Helen Gurley Brown, Germaine Greer—all warily chronicled their maturity, as of course did the writer who invented the concept of "passage," Gail Sheehy. Nora Ephron felt bad about her neck, and her anxiety spawned a best seller.

The current conversation is also informed by evolutionary biology, which evaluates traits based on their reproductive purpose. Given that menopause is non-reproductive by definition, biologists consider it a "big evolutionary puzzle," the novelist Darcey Steinke writes in her memoir, *Flash Count Diary: Menopause and the Vindication of Natural Life*. According to the prevailing view, a human female possesses all the eggs she will have while still in the womb; the number promptly begins diminishing, and by her mid-40s, the remaining ova have deteriorated. To an evolutionary biologist, this is interesting and weird. To Steinke, it was miserable and hard. Her book is lyrical but a bit depressing, because she herself was depressed.

Some women experience few symptoms during menopause, but Steinke suffered nearly two awful years of hot flashes, acute episodes that were like "four-minute surprise anxiety attacks." She sensed mortality stalking her: "For the first time, I feel I have a time stamp, an expiration date." She writes vividly and a little wistfully about sex, mourning her lost desirability, as she sees it, and the waning of her own desire. She feels angry; she yells at her husband. "Early times of sexual frenzy seem almost impossible now."

Every woman is of course entitled to—can't escape—her own response to menopause. But Steinke's melancholy reflections sound a bit retrograde, as if she can't escape those insufferable doctors, the Wilsons and the Reubens, with their pompous pronouncements about the wreckage that remains when estrogen, like a tide, drains away. "Without hormones my femininity is fraying," she writes. In a transitional state herself, she identifies with people who are transitioning out of their birth gender—not that the empathy brings much relief.

Steinke also identifies with one of the few other species that enjoy a long postmenopausal life: killer whales. In the ocean, non-reproductive females play an important role. With the wisdom of years, they guide their pod to the best salmon. Steinke kayaks in waters off the coast of Seattle, hoping to commune, and is rewarded with a magnificent breaching. "The wild matriarchs have given me hope," she writes. "They are neither frail nor apprehensive, but in every way leaders of their communities." ■

Lisa Bain's Story, Age 44

When I was 35, I had an early miscarriage. I didn't know I was pregnant but that's when I realized how irregular my periods were so the doctor referred me for blood tests and scans and it turns out my ovaries are incredibly small and the hormone results were 'catastrophic'.

I was diagnosed with the early menopause after that but my hormone results were so bad it probably started six years previously when I was diagnosed with Myelodysplastic Syndrome (MDS). Back then I had irregular periods but I didn't notice because I was too busy enjoying myself.

I was told there was absolutely no chance of falling pregnant or, if I did, carrying full-term. I was married by this point and planning a family and I was, like, what? I just couldn't believe it, couldn't take it in. All that time trying not to get pregnant to be told you can't. My husband and I were devastated and I thought he might leave but he said, 'I'm not going anywhere'. I always wanted to be a mum so to have that taken away was very hard to get my head around. The health side of things didn't bother me so much; it was the infertility.

So I had acupuncture for three months and the acupuncturist focused on my pelvic region. When I went back for blood tests I was told they were almost normal. The doctor said it could be hormone fluctuations associated with the menopause but within five months I got pregnant naturally. I didn't realize at first – we'd actually gone to Thailand to start the adoption process and a masseuse noticed I was pregnant but I didn't believe her – and so I carried on drinking. When I got home I started to feel different but still didn't believe it. Then I went for scan at 11 weeks and I was pregnant and everything was normal. I was monitored very closely because of the

MDS and went on to have a healthy baby.

After stopping breastfeeding the menopausal symptoms kicked in with a vengeance. I've now been going through them for 10 years – I've been on HRT for six years in various forms but it took 2-3 years to get the right combination. HRT needs to be regularly re-evaluated and I think my current dose needs adjusting again.

My main symptoms are that I go bright red, with sweat pouring down my face. When you sweat with the menopause you're literally drenched – it's like being cooked from the inside, like being microwaved. If I'm in a meeting I'm not afraid to say what's happening and I'll leave to cool down in the loo; I think it's better to be up front. Some days I won't have any symptoms; other days I'll get three to four hot flashes a day lasting between 1-6 minutes. They're worse now than they've ever been but I'm hoping that's a sign that things are coming to an end.

The night sweats are more of hindrance because they impact on sleep. I find that chocolate makes these worse – it could be the caffeine or sugar. Because of these and because I have fine hair I need to wash my hair every day – it sounds stupid but it's an extra thing to have to fit in on top of doing a busy job and having child to look after. My advice is grow your hair long so you can tie it back. And if you're using testosterone gel it can make you hairy so invest in a facial hair remover!

I'd also recommend being open about it – I'm the only one in my friendship group going through it but it helps to talk about it – and regular exercise is a massive benefit because of the natural endorphins it releases, which help with mood swings.

Another thing – don't accept the first thing the doctor tells you; know your own body. If the HRT you're on isn't working go back and ask for the dose to be changed.

As you go through it your thoughts and fears change such as, 'Will I keep my husband as I'm such a pain?' It's like PMS x100 but at least with PMT you know when it's coming. I feel the symptoms of the menopause all the time and now that I'm getting older I worry about thinning skin and shifting weight – I exercise as a way to counteract these things and it makes me feel better about myself but I lost my waist in my 30s, not my 50s, and there's not a thing I can do about it. Sometimes I feel resentful that I have the body of an older person – I know it sounds vain but it's part of who you are – and I'm exhausted from not sleeping. It's not much fun so the more you talk about it the better.' ■

Marisa Mazria Katz's Story

Titled: What I live with.

I'm 40. And apparently going through menopause. First came the painful sex, then came the night sweats. It started with sex. Searing, agonizing sex—just like the very first time I tried it. But now I was 40, and unlike when I was 20, there was no reason to be optimistic that the pain detonating across my pelvis would eventually go away.

I tried shifting my hips, curling onto my side, holding my breath, but each time I had sex, the throbbing pain roared. At first I was convinced it was a cyst—a ball of cells so large that nothing, barring a tampon, could enter. I had gone through five rounds of IVF to have my daughter, so it didn't seem far-fetched to concoct a theory that the injected hormones had transformed into a pulsating polyp blocking my cervix. (Though highly unlikely, it was possible.) But an excruciating 15-minute vaginal ultrasound turned up nothing.

With no apparent physical problem, I was told that I probably had **vaginismus,** a painful contraction of the muscles around the vagina that can make sex hell. According to the Cleveland Clinic, it's considered a primarily psychological condition, the pain arising from, "fear of sex, anxiety, past sexual abuse or trauma, and negative emotions towards sex." Treatment often involves therapy—but I was already in therapy and had been for years. Cracking open memories and dissecting grief in a psychotherapist's office was something I grew up with. I was flummoxed. Had I been so deep in the emotional weeds that I had unintentionally sidelined a trauma that was now wreaking havoc on my sex life? I couldn't shake the feeling that the diagnosis was a cursory reading of my pain—yet another dismissal of women's symptoms by the medical system.

And then came the sweat.

One night I awoke to a mosaic of perspiration covering my eyes, upper lip, and chest. It became my new nocturnal norm. Shirts turned sloppy wet. Waves of searing heat radiated from my core. Pajamas were ruined. The night sweats were only made worse by my almost-two-year-old deciding to transition from her bed into ours and lovingly wrapping her arms around my torso, head, or whatever she could cling to throughout the night. I felt like a human hot-water bottle.

I felt stumped by my body as it convulsed with changes I thought were meant for women much older than me. Women like my mom and my grandma. *Those* were the women who went through menopause—not new moms like me.

Finally, with a thud, my period stopped. One month turned into two, turned into eight, and I had to face facts: This looked a lot like menopause.

By this time I was only 41—a full decade younger than the **average age** of women in menopause. The idea that I might be entering **early menopause**— or even the stage before it, perimenopause—had not even been a footnote in any of the conversations I'd had with doctors up until this point. I felt stumped by my body as it convulsed with changes I thought were meant for women much older than me. Women like my mom and my grandma. *Those* were the women who went through menopause—not new moms like me.

I made an appointment with an endocrinologist, who asked me a battery of questions and then took several vials of blood. A week later he called and confirmed: I was in **perimenopause**. My ovaries were slowing down their production of estrogen until I'd never have a period again.

I thought I had years of my youth left to contemplate what this experience might mean, but my rapidly waning fertility, and even the loss of the predictable monthly routine of menstruating, forced me to face the notion that I was transitioning into the second half of my life. I felt relieved to finally have a diagnosis, but there was also a surprising feeling of shame that I had somehow hadn't managed to hold on to those precious nubile years quite as long as most women.

Unlike most of my menopausal relatives who didn't start dealing with this until their 50s, I was advised to take hormones—namely estrogen and progesterone, in the form of patches, pills, and vaginal inserts—to confront my prematurely aging body. "If you go into menopause earlier than 51, the priority in terms of medical issues we worry about is your bones," says Taraneh Shirazian, M.D., a board-certified ob-gyn and founder of **Mommy Matters**. "That is because between 40 and 51, you have that many years left ahead where the bones won't get as much estrogen."

The other main consequence of estrogen loss, I soon learned, was the vaginal dryness that was ruining my sex life. "When estrogen is decreasing, you get thinness of the vaginal walls," says Jennifer Kinder, a physical therapist and the kinesiology program director at Notre Dame de Namur University. "This decreasing can also cause vaginal dryness, which is a big one, because if a woman is dry and she wants to have sex, it can hurt."

Out of the barrage of vexing news pouring in, this was the one symptom that actually gave me a jolt of solace. All that throbbing pain wasn't in my head; it was likely a physiological response to the dip in hormones triggered by early menopause. Unfortunately, an estrogen patch wasn't going to fix it. Pelvic floor muscles (there are 14 of them down there!) tend to remember pain. "Once the pain happens, the brain protects the vaginal area with what it has: muscle tightening," says Kinder. "And when a woman attempts intercourse again, the brain remembers this and the muscles can tighten even before intercourse starts."

So I enrolled my menopausal vagina in pelvic floor therapy, which entails a physical therapist positioning her hands in various spots inside your vagina, bringing blood flow to the area and defusing spastic muscles. At first I was nonplussed—I didn't know whether to keep my eyes closed, stare at the ceiling, stay silent, or respond to the therapist's chatter (which I soon came to realize brought the extremely personal work into the realm of the mundane). I never got over the embarrassment of stripping off my pants and lying on the table while she manoeuvred inside me, but I started to understand the complexity of the area, which feels ridiculously under discussed considering how key it is to a woman during all stages of her life.

The ways women respond to menopause are just as diverse as we are—some experience nothing at all while others like yours truly undergo a torrent of transformation that can leave them feeling unrecognizable to themselves. For now, all the hormones I'm on have pushed the symptoms into a dormant state—the hot flashes have subsided, and the pain during sex has significantly waned. When I stop taking them—because the current consensus among most doctors is that hormones can work when taken in the right window but shouldn't be taken indefinitely—it's anyone's guess what will happen. The hope is that by the time the ongoing rotation of patches is finished and the last pill is swallowed, I won't be caught off guard. I'll be able to proudly say, "I was a 41-year-old menopausal woman."

In addition to my normal gynecologist, I now see one who specializes in menopause. During a recent visit she mentioned that because this process started at such a young age, I may experience a rogue period every now and again—a fleeting reminder of my more fertile youth. But for now I've grown accustomed to living without it—I never look down any more to see if I'm bleeding, and my purse no longer has the odd tampon floating around. When I think about it, what I miss most about it all is that feeling of camaraderie with my other menstruating friends—the kismet of in-sync cycles and chalking up irrational or passionate moments to "that time of the month."

I am unsurprisingly the first of my friends to go through "the change." Admittedly, it's left me feeling isolated and at times wistful for the 40s I thought I'd have. But I've also learned that menopause, just like youth, is just a word. One we honestly don't talk about nearly enough, especially considering every woman will eventually experience it. So as long as I'm going through menopause, I'm going to say it: It's a chance to calm my own sense of loss, ease others when their journey begins, and fully embrace this new chapter. ■

Isabel Gillies' Story
Titled: Early, Unexpected Menopause

It started with a miscarriage. In 2007, I was at the beginning of a spanking-new, second marriage and, thanks to a lot of happy hay rolling, I became pregnant. We loved that baby from the second after I peed on the stick. Loved it. We already had three fantastic kiddos between us, and this one would be ours. A million people would say you shouldn't name a child so early, but we couldn't help it. Billie if it was a girl, Billy if it was a boy—both for Billie Jean King. I feel a very specific tug at my heart whenever I think about him or her. I wanted to raise that baby, and I still feel like its mother.

I was more than twelve weeks along when I had the D&C miscarriage procedure. It was my third pregnancy, and I had been showing enough to make my friends squeal and give my tummy a pat. Right before they knocked me out for the procedure, my doctor leaned over and asked if I would like to know genetic information about the child. I shook my head emphatically. No. The way she said "genetic information" sounded clinical, and I hastily thought it would solely be about what had gone wrong.

We never found out the sex of the baby. I realize now not knowing anything was a mistake. I wish I knew a million things about that kid.

I would never be pregnant again.

After picking ourselves up off the floor, my husband and I started exploring fertility treatments to help get the party started. I was thirty-eight and we were still hopeful.

"Tell me about your periods," Dr. I-Will-Get-You-Pregnant asked.

I sat up a little straighter, explaining with confidence that my periods were good and robust. Not only were my periods pretty regular (sort of), but they were VERY strong and lasted for days. Huge cramps. Terrible. Like I was a teenager. Fertile, fertile, fertile.

He looked at me. I detected a hint of sympathy. "Well, what you are experiencing tells me a lot. We will do tests, but you see, when you start menstruating as a young woman, you can have heavy flow, heavy cramping, and longer periods. Then it evens out, becomes regular, and not as strong for a long time. When your body is coming closer to the end, once again, your periods become heavier, more erratic, and lengthier. It's a cycle."

I didn't like that answer, and swept it under the rug to wait to see what the results would say. The big test you take to start your fertility treatment is an FSH test. FSH is the follicle-stimulating hormone, released by the pituitary gland and located on the underside of the brain; and there is a blood test to measure those hormone levels. This is not a test given regularly to women at a routine check-up; you take it if your periods are abnormal or you're having trouble conceiving.

A week later, I was back. "I have your results," the doctor said as he walked through the door.

"Okay," I said confidently. I had always done pretty well on these kinds of tests.

"Your FSH levels are in the high sixties. Sixty-seven."

"Yeah, is that good?" (I am very dyslexic, so to me sixty-seven is a decent grade.)

"These numbers mean," he said, "it is impossible to do I.V.F. They're too high. What this signifies is that you are menopausal. You will probably soon stop getting your period. Women in their seventies have these numbers."

He was so straightforward that I felt the only thing I could do was let the steady waves of shock roll over me. There was no place in that examination room for an emotional outburst. I was silenced, but roiling inside. His words—a woman in her seventies—made my guts tangle and everything in the room turn into Claymation.

"I would advise you to see your gynecologist and start taking calcium for your bones," he said. "Without estrogen you are at risk of osteoporosis." Estrogen and bones? The information barely registered.

"So," I took in a short breath, trying to replace what had just been knocked out of me. "Is there any way for me to get pregnant? Can't you give me shots of something?" I had just been pregnant, I was in my thirties, and he was a renowned expert in this field. We were sitting in one of the most highly funded fertility clinics in the world—it couldn't be over.

"No, it would be highly unlikely for you to conceive with your eggs. There is no reversing this," he said with calm austerity.

I had assured my husband that morning that I would be fine and he could go to the office. I could have used him not only for a hand to hold, but maybe more importantly to ask more questions (his ovaries hadn't just been rendered useless), to dig deeper, to find out what this really meant— because I was dumbfounded.

"I'm in menopause? But I'm…so young."

"This is very unusual for someone your age."

I looked down at the new wedding ring on my finger and gently pushed it around.

"Am I going to, like, um…age faster?" My voice trembled. As old as he seemed to be saying I was, I felt like a five-year-old sitting on that table.

He told me no, that in all other ways, I would age normally, and then his voice turned into the teacher's voice in *Peanuts* and my imagination took me down some scary, wrinkly, decrepit, incontinent, hip-breaking, *Golden Girls* road.

With no warning, and no real understanding of menopause, I was a sleepy little town about to be smacked by a hurricane.

Here's what happened along the way to The Change. There was the pre-game show, called perimenopause, which lasted five-ish years (in hindsight, about a year of that time came before my miscarriage, which can be a sign of ensuing menopause), and blended into menopause. Some of the side effects of perimenopause and menopause were: **hot flashes** (of course); night sweats; irregular, fluttery heartbeat (I once almost called 911 while watching *Friday Night Lights* because I thought I was having a hybrid panic attack-heart attack); sudden mood swings and sudden tears (which could be unstoppable).

And that's not all…I had trouble falling asleep, trouble sleeping through the night. Irregular periods; shorter, lighter periods; heavier periods; missed periods; ten-day periods. Loss of libido. Dry vagina. Fatigue. Anxiety (oh the anxiety). There was dread, worry, doom. Depression. Difficulty concentrating, disorientation, fogginess. Memory loss——I once decided to give the kids leftover oatmeal for breakfast and in the minutes it took to heat it in the microwave, I made them pancakes, totally spacing on the oatmeal. Incontinence (no more trampolines I'm afraid). Sore old-lady joints and muscles (yoga to the rescue, but if you f-up your neck doing it like I did, then Pilates to the rescue). Breast tenderness (although my breasts got bigger, which was a plus).

Headaches. Weight gain (no amount of spinning helped). Hair loss on head and pubic area. MORE facial hair——wheeeee! Dizziness and light-headedness. Changes in body odor (sometimes weirdly for the better). Violent mood swings (more on those in a minute) and tingling in the extremities. Bleeding gums, harder time at dental cleanings, difference in breath odor from more plaque and decay. Change in vision. Osteopenia (it's bone loss, which I have in my SPINE), leading to possible osteoporosis.

AND NOBODY WARNED ME ABOUT 99 PERCENT OF IT.

Even though the doctor did tell me I had the hormone levels of a septuagenarian, I was in denial about my waning fertility and what accompanied this change. Initially, the only side effect I actually attributed to menopause was the clichéd hot flashes. My first massive attack came in a restaurant when I was having lunch with a friend. It was February, two months after my miscarriage. I wanted to rip off my t-shirt in the middle of the Mercer Hotel dining room (but settled for whipping my hair into a ponytail). My friend was wearing a lavender sweater set—perfectly comfortable. A hot flash is not like when you are sweating from a jog, or because it's 87 degrees out. It came out of nowhere, and felt like every pore on my body was instantaneously producing pencil-dot sized beads of perspiration, from my scalp to my shins. Night sweats and hot flashes began to disrupt my life—I woke up in a drenched nightgown and sheets regularly for the next year. Clearly not great, but you can live with them.

A more perplexing turn of events, and a definite bummer, was my loss of sex drive. I was madly in love and had just gotten married; there was no reason for me to have a "whatever" relationship to sex. I half-heartedly assured myself it was okay to not feel like a twenty-year-old 24/7. After all, many of my friends who were nearing a decade of marriage were telling tales of things cooling in the bedroom—I lumped myself in with them.

What tipped me off that my loss of sex drive had nothing to do with my husband: The following summer, about eighteen months after the D&C, I went to Maine with the kids while Peter stayed in New York. We didn't see each other for three weeks—and I didn't masturbate. What red-blooded American female does that? One in menopause. The doctor had said something about upping my calcium intake, but didn't mention losing serious boudoir mojo. The scientific term for it is—vaginal atrophy. You can see why people don't talk about this stuff—but please, let's get over it.

By an order of magnitude, the worst part of menopause was my erratic temper. For two years, I was as easy to set off as a mousetrap—and it could come down as hard. Typically, when women go through menopause, their children are college-aged and on their own. Mine were in elementary school and living in my house during all of this upheaval. Without warning, I could experience melancholy so deep I would cry until I looked like Rocky Balboa after a run in with Apollo Creed's right hook. I tried to keep the emotional hurricane away from my family, but I was at its mercy, didn't know when it would sweep through me, and sometimes they were directly in its path. I once got so upset with my husband (for something unmemorable and trivial), I tore our up our wedding album. I knew in the back of my mind that I'd made it on iPhoto and could print another one in the morning, which I did, but it was all so dark. I was out of control. (Just ask my kids.) Sometimes I would look out onto the Hudson River from my bedroom, and feel like sinking to the bottom.

I also wasn't sleeping. Up until that time in my life a solid eight or even ten hours a night was absolutely no problem, but when I was in menopause, getting to sleep was unachievable.

With all the anger, sadness and insomnia, I thought I was having a breakdown, I felt helpless. I remember looking into Peter's face after a particularly bad crying fit and he said, kindly, "It's like you're unhinged." A little less than two years had passed since the D&C. I was not associating my behavior with anything physical. I went to a psychiatrist, but I never told him I was in menopause, or made mention of a miscarriage—as clear as it is now, it didn't click that my behavior was all the result of hormonal changes to my body. I'm the kind of girl who went to the gym when I had cramps and rolled my eyes at friends kvetching about their PMS. If I was acting bonkers, I thought it wasn't because of "women's issues," it was because I was becoming insane. My therapist gave me tools to help me with the depression and temper, but without the physical piece of the puzzle, he was at a disadvantage.

You're considered in menopause when you haven't had a period for twelve months. I stopped getting my period altogether about three to four years after my miscarriage. Just after that time, I went back to the same psychiatrist after a particularly steady and happy summer—I was feeling…normal…and trying to figure out why. He asked me what had changed and it was only then I told him that a doctor years ago had given me the diagnosis of early ovarian failure when I had a miscarriage. His face dropped: If only he had known. It was then, after the storm had cleared, that the dots were more, neatly, connected, that I linked all my physical symptoms and mental behavior to menopause, and figured out how to feel like my (new) self.

Today, I have three teens in the house and it ain't nothing but a thing. I never cry uncontrollably in the bathroom, my husband and I once again make love not war (with the help of understanding and coconut oil), and I feel peaceful, much more like a dove than a grenade. I take estrogen, and that's because I have no history of ovarian, uterine, or breast cancer in my family. But the estrogen prescription might change as soon as my next doctor appointment. What I learned about mitigating menopausal symptoms is that you have to be flexible, investigative, and preferably prepared for some explorations to go askew.

Soon after the fertility doctor told me I was barren, I had sought out an Ayurvedic doctor in New York. I thought even if the white coats are singing one tune, there is a whole lot of music out there. The Ayurvedic doctor only had to lift up the skin on my hand and let it go to tell that my FSH hormone levels were skyrocketing (menopause causes loss of plasticity in the skin). Just as the other doctor had said, this doctor didn't think she could help me conceive or reverse Mother Nature's plans, but she could give me herbs to take that "may help." In my desperation and urgency to find the miracle, I rushed home and swallowed all the herbs she prescribed while standing at my kitchen counter. I'm not sure I even read the directions. (Yes, I wonder now if I took more than what was necessary.) I looked like Lucy in the factory trying to eat the chocolates.

And, as if I were in a Nora Ephron movie, that night I had a twentieth high school reunion dinner—you know, the gathering where you really want to have your shit together and look "better than you did in high school!" Even if a twentieth reunion sounds old to some, it wouldn't be unheard of for a classmate to be pregnant at one—I wanted so badly to be one of those women.

Sometime between gobbling down pill after pill (I couldn't tell you now what the herbs were) and standing-around-talking-about-jobs-and-spouses-with-a-glass-of-chardonnay, I had an outlandish allergic reaction. By the time I had gone through the buffet line, my face resembled a pink, cream-filled snowball, and my ear lobes were grapes. I was itchy even under my armpits. I sat down on a sofa, plate on lap, searching for words to explain to my classmates—most of whom I hadn't seen since high school—what was happening.

I threw in the towel: "I'm having an allergic reaction to a field-full of Ayurvedic herbs I ate today because I'm in"—I don't think I'd ever uttered the words in public—"early menopause."

Someone hilariously and instantly said, "God that sucks."

And it does! It does suck.

But you can also kind of get into it. Remember this all happened extremely early for me, so it took years to figure out, but once I had embraced and gotten woke to the irreversible changes in my body, I stopped fighting and started honoring the truth. Not only did I start to get behind myself as a maturing woman, but I figured out fun stuff to do. I could slather oil all over my skin three times a day and not break out. I had a ball researching every essential oil under the sun. I even wrote an article about essential oils for *Cosmo*—a job that felt sexier than any job I had when I was menstruating.

Not long ago, a younger friend was a little discouraging when I told her I was writing about menopause. "But it will feel like this huge nightmare coming at you," she said, her hands shooting up in the air like she was about to block a Frisbee careening toward her head. "Who will want to read it?" Her barely-thirty-year-old forehead wrinkled with concern.

I guess she is right—it isn't the same as cracking open *Are You There God? It's Me Margaret.* before you got your period. Nor is it putting a pillow under your shirt to see what you will look like pregnant. But I believe that knowing what it could be like is better than not knowing. And starting to wrap your head around what our bodies will do is as important as tucking a tampon in your evening purse. It's better to be prepared.

It's been ten years since my miscarriage. When I look back, I see a young woman, scrambling, rollercoastering, and ignorant. Today, clarity and knowledge feel necessary to me, so I listen carefully and try to own what is real. Just last week my Chinese medicine doctor, Jane Seymour Page, M.Sc., L.Ac., said this:

"In Chinese Medicine the seasons of life are respected and celebrated for what they are; varied interpretations of, capacities for, and choices about the use of energy. Each season has its own limitations and opportunities. For most women, once fertility has waned, then ceased, the libido ultimately decreases and the tissues change. There is an option to shift focus inward and plumb the depths of wisdom earned; to experience and participate in life with authority. This does not imply that sexual activity disappears, it simply calls for a slower, richer, less frequent participation. We then have energy to expend on as yet unexplored aspects of life. Forcing youthful demands on an evolving elder is foolish and absurd because it runs counter to their purpose. Whether we have raised children or not, whether we have partnered with another or not, this is a time to give the self primacy and to interface with our communities with warmth and discretion."

I wish someone had laid that on me back when.

Menopause is hard, there is no question, but there is no reason to think all is lost. There is a ton you can do for the sad, shadowy feelings (shrinks, walks, community engagement, friends, music, sex), dryness (argan oil, coconut oil, hormone replacement therapy, longer-more-deeply-engaged-sex), insomnia (magnesium, exercise, reading, meditation, sex) mind fog (word retrieval problems, humor). I've tried a lot, some of it works, some doesn't. But you can't do anything about perimenopause or menopause if you don't know what it is, and why it's happening. So, let's talk—to mothers, doctors of all kinds, older pals, husbands, wives, partners, each other.

The big feelings I was getting through perimenopause and menopause, however scary and disruptive, were like the unknown side of the universe. There were frightening moments of darkness, but also bright, unexpected comets (I wrote three books in the last ten years), towering and then plummeting climates, and different speeds of light. I learned how deep we can go, how much we can feel, and how mysterious it all is. I also learned, once again, how grateful I am for people sticking by me when humanity roars.

The scientist Carl Sagan said my favorite quote of all time, "In the cosmos, there is no refuge from change." Is that true or what? Goodness, all I have to do is look at the teenagers in my apartment to see Carl knew of what he spoke. For me, now that my hormones have balanced, I recognize myself once again—I feel normal, and it's a mighty relief. But I'm staying alert, I'm on my toes, I'm open to what might, or what certainly will change in the great, wide future. ▪

Anonymous Story
Titled: All Changed

"Oh for fuck's sake, why can't they design kitchen equipment that does what it's supposed to do? This is FUCKING RIDICULOUS!"

Other family members looked on nervously as I flung things round the kitchen. The trigger event for this Gordon Ramsay style kitchen meltdown? While draining pasta, a few strands of spaghetti had slipped through the colander into the sink. I know, terrible isn't it? I blame my hormones for the extreme reaction.

Until about two years ago I had only a vague notion of what the menopause entailed. I knew about the night sweats and hot flushes, but that was about it. Menopause is deemed to have happened when you have gone 12 months without a period. What I now know is that when you reach this milestone, all the drama is over. Perimenopause is where it's really at. Perimenopause is the term for the fun-filled years leading up to the menopause, and it lasts on average for four or five years. It's been quite an adventure so far.......

It all started innocently enough with irregular but otherwise normal periods. This is grand, I thought to myself. Then last summer, the famous hot flushes and night sweats kicked in, but that stage didn't last very long. Still grand. Though given the unpredictable nature of perimenopause, I suppose they might be back (great!). In the last 8 months or so I've experienced a range of other, more annoying symptoms.

Menopause brain
This my term for the brain fog, lack of concentration and mental confusion which can mark perimenopause and which at times has caused me to question my sanity. I've always been absent minded but this is on a whole new level. Stress exacerbates these symptoms hugely. During a recent family crisis I found myself making really stupid mistakes at work. I remember being horrified on seeing a cash reconciliation sheet which was clearly the work of an innumerate idiot, only to realize the idiot was me – I'd been handling payments that day.

Long hunts for the car in car parks are a regular occurrence, as I have no recollection whatsoever of parking the thing. Worst of all was was a two month long 'reader's block' where I found myself incapable of concentrating enough to read a book. Tragic. I made my excuses at the book club.

Menopause narcolepsy

In the last few months I've learned that if I want to achieve anything after about 4pm on any given day, I need to keep away from soft furniture. If my ass lands on a sofa or bed, however briefly, I WILL fall asleep. Instantly and deeply. The fatigue is extreme and overwhelming. There are also occasional spells of dizziness and light-headedness where, like a posh Victorian lady, I've had an attack of the vapors necessitating a little sit down because I feel weak. Smelling salts please!

Rivers of blood (You have been warned)

Anyway, last week I finally copped that there's probably a cause and effect connection between the rivers of blood, the tiredness and the brain fog. I dragged myself off to the GP. Sure enough, blood tests showed that I'm anaemic so a course of iron and B12 injections should sort that out. As for the periods from hell? "You can't put up with that" declared the doctor, making me want to kiss her (I didn't). She's packing me off to a gynaecologist to see what can be done to resolve matters.

Every woman will experience perimenopause differently of course. My own mother says that her periods just stopped in her 50s and she had no symptoms in the lead-up (my mother is what's known as a trooper). I decided to write this blog post to share my experience as I've found that it's still a fairly taboo subject here in prudish Ireland. Although I've recently discovered a website called "My Second Spring" which is a good outlet for women going through *adopts Les Dawson mother-in-law expression* 'The Change'. ■

Angela's Story

I can't recall the exact moment I first said the M word out loud. But I am sure it was waaaay before the event itself. And I'd say it had a smug tone to it. You see, a lifelong practitioner of the 5 and 10 year plans, I had already scoped out in my early 40s what 50 and the inevitable arrival of Menopause was going to look like for me. With the naiveté of the ignorant (or was it arrogant?) I just *knew* my midlife rite of passage was going to be dynamic, feisty, and fabulous. Hell, it was Celtic Tiger Ireland. We were all unstoppable….then….Menopause: ahead of schedule.

Fast-forward a few years from that date. My menopausal moment had arrived, earlier than scheduled. Sooner than planned, I thought, but, with plenty of change under my belt in the intervening years – late motherhood, moving country, mothballing a career, "the change" would be a walk in the park. Heck, I was practically an expert.

Except that it wasn't. It was a rollercoaster. Dips, swings, loop the loops. The sleep deprivation of the baby years gave way to even more punishing night sweats and chills. In the dead of night, anxiety came calling, churning the slightest ache or pain into the possibility of serious, life threatening illnesses. Every morning, I woke to find my mood on the floor, and my energy levels not much higher. Daylight brought a different type of thermostat malfunction - sudden rushes of unsettling, humid heat and random explosions of irrational irritation. . So far, so very *un*-fabulous. So not me! my younger self would have thought. The unremitting cycle of tiredness triggering sugar cravings, spurring ever-hotter flashes, followed by sugar crashes was close to unbearable. I was, as my American sisters would put it, a hot mess. Advice was scant. Take off a sweater, a relative in her late sixties suggested, echoing the widespread mantra of the middle aged magazines to "Dress in layers." (She had a faint recollection of getting a bit warm in meetings sometimes.) No one offered advice on how to manage the inconvenience of multiple showers and clothing changes a day – not to mention the extra laundry duty that comes with it.

I stuck it out for almost two years, more from helplessness than grit, before seeking help from Dr Rachel Mackey at the Women's Health Clinic in Dun Laoighaire. A specialist in menopause, with a published women's health book covering the subject, she surely could help. I knew from my 3am digital expeditions that hormone balancing therapy - what used to be called HRT - was a no no for someone with a family history of breast cancer. I also knew, though, having happened upon the infamous and ominous sounding 34 Signs of Menopause website, that I'd only experienced a few of the delights of menopause thus far. More fun in prospect – it seemed time to call in the SWAT team.

Ageing overnight. I'm almost embarrassed to admit it, but it was vanity that eventually took me to Dr Rachel's door. (That, and a plummeting libido.) The face in the mirror looked like the older sister I'd never had, and she seemed to show up overnight. My skin, hair, nails, body, all seemed to undergo a series of stealthy little losses that added up to quite radical change. Weight crept on in places it never settled before- something I'd managed to avoid without too much effort for the best part of half a century. Nails weakened, hair coarsened - and migrated to my face. Grooves deepened, pores widened, skin folded and sagged a little bit more. It seemed downright ungrateful to complain about such minor cosmetic sacrifices when women in the last century would have considered themselves lucky to live to a menopausal age in a state of relative health.

Still, the cumulative toll of sweating and sleep deficit, a hollowed face and a filled out middle, a lower mood and a higher level of anxiety can be devastating to a woman's self esteem, especially in a world where ageing is regarded as an aberration and 50 is expected to be the new 40.

Time has passed and I've at last settled into an accommodation with my post menopausal body and the pattern of a hormonally volatile day. Dr Rachel introduced me to the wonder of Sylk lubricant which slowly took effect. As for the rest, I'm a slow learner but I'm getting there. I know that the humble little polo mint can prompt a ferocious hot flash. (And that it can be a handy heat source on a winter's morning). So too, a particularly strong cup of coffee. A glass of prosecco. Green and Black's chocolate. A good giggle. All of the best things in life seem to spark the familiar surge in body temperature. I know what fabrics overheat me – most synthetics – and think ahead to the rooms and venues I might find myself in and plan strategic exit points. I get the sleep I can, to reign in sugar cravings. I take considerable comfort from the upbeat, smart, capable women I've met recently who can turn their transition into a positive opportunity.

I try to exercise, because I absolutely know it's the one prescription that works for women my age – on so many levels, from protecting bone health to keeping depression at bay - but I've got a way to go. My weight remains somewhat stable, although I am still mourning my pre-change body, which managed to come through two pregnancies and four decades relatively unscathed, but has succumbed to some serious hormonal shape shifting. Bikinis are now well beyond me, while burkas and chadors are starting to look very appealing - and in that there's the start of relinquishing youthful things.

Letting go can be liberating, But giving up those things that defined your younger self can be a fiercely liberating thing, You do let yourself go a little, as the cliché goes, but in the best possible way. You still aim for a groomed exterior but increasingly don't give a hoot who thinks you look good or not. Ditto your clothes.

The opinion that matters most post-menopause is yours. And that's empowering. What's inside becomes more important than what's on the surface – when you realise that the real power source is no longer physical attractiveness but character and experience. Change really doesn't faze you any more – you've navigated hormone hell and all the indignities that go with it and whatever's coming next, you'll work it out and you're pretty sure you'll be grand. ■

MENOPAUSE: SEVEN STORIES BY JENNIFER MURCH

At a friend's 50th birthday celebration this summer, a bunch of us were standing around the campfire when I hissed at the birthday girl, "Hey, do you still have your period?"

And just like that, we were all firing questions at each other: What are *your* symptoms? Do you have more energy now that you're no longer bleeding? Did your periods get heavier towards the end? And, what, exactly, *is* the difference between perimenopause and menopause anyway?

It was so weird, we all agreed. Here we were, a bunch of grown-ass women yet we knew next to nothing about this big physical change our bodies were beginning to go through.

It's because no one talks about it, we decided. Everybody talks about getting your period or getting pregnant — that's easy; it's so *obvious* — but since menopause is a gradual shift, and messy and complicated to boot, it's often not until women are on the other side looking back that we begin to comprehend what we just went through. Or at least that's how it *feels* to those of us who are perimenopausal. Now, we bleed. Then, we won't. WHAT HAPPENS IN BETWEEN???

So I sent emails to a bunch of women asking them to pretty please share what menopause was like for them. As the responses came in, I was surprised by how many of the women discredited their experiences. *Oh, my menopause was medically-induced,* they said. Or, *It was really confusing because I was going through other stuff at the same time.* It was almost as though they thought that, if their experience deviated from textbook menopause, then it didn't count.

"But it's the complicated and confusing experiences that we [perimenopausal women] especially need to hear," I told one friend who felt like her experience was too much of an exception to be helpful. "The greater the variety, the better we can manage our expectations."

Besides, textbook menopause (which, to me, is: turn fifty, periods taper off, hot flashes and mood swings, then, BAM, done) was too simplistic, too narrow. I craved the stories, the *real* women sharing the details of what menopause was actually *like.*

So here is my attempt at getting the conversation started: seven women, seven stories. Many thanks to the women for taking the time to share with us! (All names have been changed to protect privacy.)

A final note on terminology (which I had to look up, and even then I got it half wrong and had to be corrected): *premenopausal women* can reproduce, *perimenopausal women* are in the process of losing their ability to reproduce (this can last 10-15 years), *menopausal* women can no longer reproduce — a woman is considered menopausal when she's not had a period for twelve months, but she's *in* menopause during that year-ish — and *postmenopausal* women are, well, done with menopause entirely, though some symptoms do linger, I'm learning.

Meet the Women

Rachel, 57

I have no idea when I started menopause, how long it lasted, or when it ended. I had a hysterectomy at age 42. My uterus was removed, due to fast-growing, grapefruit-sized benign tumor, but my ovaries remained — the idea was that they would still do what they do, hormone-wise, I guess. I stopped having periods immediately, obviously, so I lost that gauge on what was happening with my body.

Sarah, 77

I started perimenopause in my 40's and it lasted for 10 years. When I was about 50, I started having very heavy periods and had several D&C's, which would help for awhile and then the heavy bleeding would start up again. I remember having a period for six weeks before one of the D&C's. Everything quit at age 55.

Rosanna, 65

I was about 50 when my periods started to become less predictable. This was not normal, so I knew something was changing. At 53, I had one very heavy period (while we were out of town at a wedding, of all places!), and then after that they were more irregular. Then, just before I turned 55, we had a traumatic life event and I never had another period. That was the end of that.

Nancy, 72

By age 34 or so, I could no longer reproduce like a rabbit — conceiving our youngest took a year. Then, at around age 36, pregnant again, I spontaneously aborted. This was expected, since I'd been told I had a low progesterone count and hadn't felt inclined to interfere with nature by taking hormones. I don't remember when I reached menopause.

Liz, 60

I was 41½ when I noticed a change in my periods. I'd just stopped nursing my youngest, but I don't think that had anything to do with it. My periods had never been clockwork regular, but I noticed they became increasingly irregular over the next couple years. It's hard to remember exactly when I stopped; I just continued to go longer and longer between periods. In the end, I hadn't had a period for six months, and then I had the mother-of-all-heavy-periods. That was the last one! I remember telling my sister about it; she'd experienced the very same thing, with the very same timing.

Leslie, 72

My hysterectomy was so sudden and so completely unexpected that it was as detrimental to my mental health as any of the other extreme medical procedures that I've had, and there have been a few. Part of this is due to the fact that I had no time to even consider the procedure. I was at the hospital, prepped for a hysteroscopy — a procedure where, as I understood, they'd simply look at the uterus — when the doctor casually suggested that he might do a hysterectomy if he saw lots of endometrial tissue adhered to the uterus. If so, what did I want him to do with my ovaries? I paused a bit, and then replied, "Oh, just take them out. They won't be functioning much longer anyway. I don't want to wake up and find that I need another surgery!" So, you see. I have my own ignorance for some of the blame. When I came out of surgery, I learned that the doctor had cleaned me out. One ovary was adhered to my uterus. The other he just took because it was easy to do.

Karla, 53

I don't recall a specific start time to all the changes. It was so gradual, the slow drip of the water. No day to pinpoint, but maybe I'm just not remembering it…. maybe it started four years ago? I think my first realization was a spotty menstrual cycle, but since my cycle wasn't ever really bad, I didn't pay attention until I had my annual midwife visit and she started asking questions. She commented that I could be in perimenopause, which I'd never heard of. So there's that! After that, I paid attention a little more.

***

Symptoms

Rachel: Four to five years after my hysterectomy, I had a "breakdown" of sorts: a very difficult period of insomnia, depression, anxiety, unexplained weight loss, zero libido, frequent crying. One night I ended up in the ER with chest pain that ultimately was called anxiety. In hindsight, I can see I was doing more than was healthy in terms of a stressful job (and there were unusual stresses at work). I felt like, and maybe was, a horrible mother.

Sarah: Perimenopause hit me as extreme anxiety and insomnia. I would go night after night with no sleep at all while teaching full time. I also started having night sweats (but not very many hot flashes during the day). Because of the lack of sleep, I started having depression, weight loss, and, because I was always tired, I didn't want to go anywhere, except for my job. I was also parenting a teenager who was into partying and drinking, which contributed to my anxiety.

Rosanna: I must not have had many symptoms because I really don't remember drastic changes. I started having hot flashes in my early 50's — they were almost welcome because I have always been cold. (When I was younger, I couldn't wait for menopause so I could maybe be warm; alas, it's a different kind of heat and has not solved my problem of being cold. I hate winter!) I remember going through a phase where I could not wait for the hot flashes to be done, but I don't think that lasted much longer than a year.

Nancy: No problems. Nothing like many other women's crazy-making experiences.

Liz: I had hot flashes off and on, but I wouldn't say they were very severe. Through the whole experience, I kind of felt like I was someone else. I can't quite explain the feeling — kind of jumpy inside, and I found it hard to focus. That went on for quite a few years until I felt more calm and focused.

Leslie: Right away I had terrible night sweats and panic attacks. Another very definite consequence: drying up. I noticed my hair changed texture, my skin lost some of its elasticity, and I started using drops in my eyes for "dry eye." On the plus side, there were no more odd pains in various parts of my body — migraine and leg aches — that, in retrospect probably were connected to endometriosis, the disease I probably had and that no one ever mentioned.

Karla: The absolute most frustrating thing for me (besides a decrease in libido) has been memory loss and forgetfulness. It feels like it snuck up on me, which made me feel like I was losing it. I've had moments of crazy thoughts of thinking I had Alzheimer's. I don't remember some "obvious" events from just the year before — it's become a family joke. And really, is this just aging or is it all connected to perimenopause? I say that because, around the same time, my eyesight started to go, I felt like I only had to *look* at food to gain weight, and I developed the ability to predict weather through my aging knee. Also, I started having hot flashes at night, I began constantly asking my kids to repeat things, my hair began greying, there was more hair on my chin, I started having hot flashes *during* the day and times I had higher-than-normal levels of anxiety.

***

Coping Mechanisms

Rachel: I tried everything: exercise, eating right, supplements, prayer, mediation, massage, consultation with a natural healer, cognitive behavioral counseling, medication. Somewhere in there, a nurse practitioner suggested HRT (hormonal replacement therapy), which I did. I lost track of how long I was on Estradiol — I just took it to help with everything: insomnia, moods, libido. In recent years, a nurse practitioner suggested it might be time to stop since I'd been on it for ten years.

Sarah: My doctor put me on a hormone replacement regimen, which wasn't very helpful, so then he put me on a depression medicine. I put on a happy mask when I was out with people, and very few friends knew what I was dealing with.

Rosanna: When I realized that regular coffee made my hot flashes worse, I started making either full or half decaf and that seemed to help.

Leslie: The doctor immediately offered a prescription for fake estrogen, but I refused since I was already phobic about blood clots.

Karla: Talking to women friends: the most valuable resource to be found. Exercise is now more for mental health than physical health. Also, I lasered my facial hair, I began to move to the couch when my husband started snoring (sleep is not overrated), and I bit the bullet and joined a weight loss program.

***

Relationships and Sex

Rachel: During menopause, my marriage was extremely strained. Was my marriage strained because I was depressed/menopausal? Or was I depressed and desperate because my marriage was crap? Chicken and egg. Who knows.

Sarah: I didn't share my problems with my female work colleagues, since many of them were younger than me. My husband was kind, but not a great support, as men just don't understand.

Rosanna: Funny you should mention sex! Again, it is one of those things that nobody talks about but I am really curious, too. I have very little to no sex drive and it has been that way ever since that traumatic life event. I'm not sure if the trauma brought that on, or if it was menopause. I think the changes in our relationship may be been partially on account of menopause, but I also think that it is much more complex than that. So much in our everyday lives has also changed as we are getting older, and that factors in big time!

Nancy: My husband still thinks I'm the cat's meow. But sex takes a lot of patience and kindness. It just doesn't seem important. It's not something I think much about. Those hormones aren't driving me. No libido.

Liz: I don't feel the desire for sex that I had in my younger years. That was the only downside to the whole process.

Leslie: As well as all the other drying up, my vaginal area dried up as well. All you women who are about to have your uterus removed, take note: Sex will never yield quite the same degree of pleasure, as you will no longer have a contracting organ in there to "move mountains" for you (so to speak).

Karla: There's definitely a decrease in libido. It is hard to be the instigator when it's lost its fun. I feel guilty for making him be the initiator so I am trying to be more intentional, which totally takes the fun out of it. I'm still learning to communicate better about this and be truthful and honest. I'm also still happily married and feel grateful for my main squeeze. I do put up with a lot — but he probably puts up with more.

***

Looking back, any insights? How do you feel now?

Rachel: I didn't ask women much about this when it was going on. Looking back, I think it was pretty much survival time. Maybe more conversations with women who were 10 or 15 years older would have helped. Also, I notice when I am hating myself and try to reframe my thinking. For example, I hate my feet. They are ugly — not cute in sandals. But I try to switch those thoughts to appreciation that I can walk and run and hike and bike. I like the concept of referring to my body as "she" rather than "it."

Sarah: I was so thankful when I was in my 50's and felt normal again!

Rosanna: I can't say that menopause has made me feel different physically, but it has affected my metabolism. I try to walk 1-2 miles several days a week since my work is pretty sedentary, but I still struggle with weight gain.

Nancy: I don't mourn the changes. I still feel womanly.

Liz: Now that it's all over I feel really good. No more emotional ups and downs. No more of that monthly bloated feeling. No more worries about when the next period would come. And I have lots of energy.

Leslie: I realize I've focused more on the cataclysmic nature of my menopausal experience, and I often feel bitter about the perhaps ten more years I might have had at least one functioning ovary (I have no idea if there are other treatments for endometriosis now, or even at the time), but my advice is: Hang onto *all* your female organs as long as possible!! And TALK, TALK, TALK to your doctor — nowadays perhaps a woman.

Wow, unheard of in the day! — about each and every detail of every aspect of what they suggest. Also, *ask* about prescriptions and other solutions to deal with whatever it is you're experiencing.

Karla: I finally paid the money and joined **Noom**. I was so tired of doing all the right things and not losing weight, but, like a good Mennonite, I hated to pay for it. So I vowed to do exactly what they said so for the first 3 months so I could quit and not pay more. And it worked! I lost what I hoped to and have kept it off for six months. This has made me feel more confident and feel better about myself. I'm so glad I did it and I feel like my weight is back to where it was before having kids. Additionally, other things that I have noticed and am grappling with are more facial wrinkles and hair, loose skin, and wiry white hair. I'd like to say that I'm slowly accepting these things, but I'll probably be working on this for the rest of my life. I'm such a work in progress. ■

The Bitch Is Back *By Sandra Tsing Loh*

Are menopausal women mad, bad, and dangerous? Yes—but they're really just returning to normal.

DURING MENOPAUSE, *a* woman can feel like the only way she can continue to exist for 10 more seconds inside her crawling, burning skin is to walk screaming into the sea—grandly, epically, and terrifyingly, like a 15-foot-tall Greek tragic figure wearing a giant, pop-eyed wooden mask. Or she may remain in the kitchen and begin hurling objects at her family: telephones, coffee cups, plates. Or, as my mother did in the 1970s, she may just eerily disappear into her bedroom, like a tide washing out—curtains drawn, door locked, dead to the world, for days, weeks, months (some moms went silent for years). Oh, for a tribal cauldron to dive into, a harvest moon to howl at, or even an online service that provides—here's an idea!—demon gypsy lovers.

But no, this is 21st-century America, so there is no ancient womyn's magic for us but rather, as usual for female passages, a stack of medically themed self-help books. (I ask you: Where are the vampire novels for perimenopausal women? Werewolf tales? Pirate movies?) That's right—to fully get our crone on, we're supposed to *read*, even though it may feel, what with the giant Greek chthonic headpiece, that one can barely see out the eyeholes. (Who can focus on words on a page? Who can even remember where she left her giant octagonal Medea-size reading glasses?) Rest assured, though: I'm here to help. Gentle reader, if you are a female of transitional age, which can apparently be anywhere from 35 to 65 these days, let me be your Virgil to the literature of menopause. Long have I wandered through the dry riverbeds, long have I suffered; now I've come back to share my wisdom.

To set the stage, here is a selection of titles from my local bookstore's women's section: *Could It Be … Perimenopause?*; *Before Your Time: The Early Menopause Survival Guide*; *The Natural Menopause Plan*; *Second Spring*; *Menopause Reset!: Reverse Weight Gain, Speed Fat Loss, and Get Your Body Back in 3 Simple Steps*; and the slightly ominously titled *What Nurses Know … Menopause* (two words: *atrophic vaginitis*). On the cover of a typical menopause book, instead of the perhaps more to-the-point fanged woman with the Medusa do, one is far more likely to see a lone flower—a poppy, perhaps a daisy. Curious choice? Well, no, because as one begins to read the war stories of the M.D., Ph.D., and R.N. (atrophic vaginitis!) authors who dominate this genre, one sees narratives that are indeed Stuart Smalley–esque. Here's a pastiche:

Mary Anne, age 48, came into my office feeling overweight and bloated. She hadn't been sleeping, work was stressful, her husband had just gone on disability, and he required daily care. Mary Anne complained to me of lower-back problems and gastritis, and also cramping during sex, which had become more and more infrequent. She was extremely depressed about moving her 84-year-old mother to a nursing home, and upon examination I noticed vaginal inflammation.

As unappetizing as that just was to read, be glad you saw only one such passage—I must have read a hundred. Because clearly, from the medical-professional point of view, menopause, or really the run-up to it called perimenopause, is a parade of baleful, bloated middle-aged women ("Lisa, 52," "Carolyn, 47," "Suzanne, 61") trudging into their doctors' offices complaining of lower-back pain and family care-giving issues and diminished libidos and personal dryness and corns. As they sit wanly on the tables in their paper gowns, they arduously count out their irregular periods—from 35 days to 44 days to 57, going heavy to light, light to heavy, sometimes with spotting, sometimes with flooding, sometimes flood-spotting, sometimes spot-flooding. Why this variation? So easy to understand, really. The simple science: ovarian production of the estrogens and progesterone becomes erratic during perimenopause, with unpredictable fluctuations in levels, which in turn can result in many different symptoms, including major mood swings. But sometimes not. You may never feel any of this! Because here's the key: *All women are different.*

And yet, even though we all are different, the list of prescriptions for us seems to be very much the same, and none of its fun. If one *must* tinker with hormone-replacement therapy, one may—briefly, in moderation. But from this point on, The Change is about healthy lifestyle. We're all to get more exercise, drink more water, do yoga stretches before bed, cut out alcohol and caffeine, and yet (and how does this follow?) reduce stress. Even the flirty exhortations to have more sex feel like yet another job on life's chore wheel (given that it's supposed to be with your mate of 20 years rather than with Johnny Depp). And don't forget all the deep sensory pleasures of a reduced-calorie diet. *Menopause Reset!* at least initially seemed to promise a nutritional miracle cure for that mysterious spare beach floaty that arrives after 40. I for one was excited to see that, instead of *Black Swan*–ing it until dinner, as apparently so many of us women do (in order to heap our measly 1,500 calories together into one meal a person might actually want to eat), you're supposed to eat many tiny meals constantly. Hurray! But alas, after reading much dietary advice for menopausal women, I concluded that, in the horrible new metrics of midlife, each of the following constitutes a *meal*:

Meal No. 1 (8 a.m.):
2 tsp. non-fat yogurt

Meal No. 2 (10 a.m.):
3 almonds (unsalted)

Meal No. 3 (12 p.m.)
2 oz. low-fat barley soufflé (see Appendix D)

Meal No. 4 (2 p.m.)
small Bell pepper
1 tsp. flaxseed

Just staying *awake* all day to *eat* the food—while of course getting in those 15 reps an hour of sex with your 50-something husband—seems a challenge. No wine, though: best to pair vaginal dryness with buckwheat tempeh. Oh! Oh! Oh! Where is the plate-glass window to hurl phone through? Why is life worth living? Ouch, my corns!

SO THAT'S THE basic physiological landscape of menopause. Dry as the riverbeds can seem, though, one menopause book does rise like Mount Etna above the rest. Now celebrating its 10th anniversary, it is the bible of middle-aged womanhood: *The Wisdom of Menopause*, by Christiane Northrup, M.D. Having recently spent (20? 50? 80?) hours with it, I've come to believe that *The Wisdom of Menopause* is a masterwork. Weighing in at two pounds and 656 pages, it is an astonishingly complete, mind-bogglingly detailed orrery of the achingly complex, wheels-and-dials-filled Ptolemaic universe that is Womanhood. Featuring, arch-conventionally, its smiling doctor/author on a soothing pastel cover, the book is very much of the genre, and yet explodes it. Northrup presents both a celebration of Western medical practice and a revolt against it. Three times as big as the others, *Wisdom* is no less than the Jupiter in the menopause-book solar system, our *Gravity's Rainbow*.

Let me now gloriously unbutton my too-tight mom jeans, wave my Hadassah arms (even more hideous term heard recently—*bat wings*), and wax on. Are you grasping, yet, the scope of this thing? *Wisdom* is a Homeric poem of modern femalehood. No stone from Western or Eastern (or Southern or Northern) medicine is left unturned, from folic acid to breast exams to personal dancing to selenium to feng shui to cosmetic surgery (Northrup allows it, while counseling discretion as a protection against judgmental friends). Woo-woo passages on Motherpeace Tarot cards and the chakra work of the astrologer Barbara Hand Clow alternate with biological analyses of an almost kidney-squeezing complexity. Which is not to say there isn't tons of news you can use:

I highly recommend a snack at around four in the afternoon, right during the time when blood sugar, mood, and serotonin tend to plummet.

This totally hit home. Although the Hour of the Wolf is typically considered 4 o'clock in the morning, for many mothers of school-age children, how many of our inner wolves appear at afternoon carpool time?

Even Suze Orman makes a guest appearance, in a TV green room (the place where all modern witches gather):

She told me that you can see people's ill health in their money and cash flow first because money has nowhere to hide an energy imbalance.

You either have positive cash flow or you have debt. Simple. Sooner or later, if the behavior patterns and beliefs that create money problems are not addressed, they will manifest as health problems in the body.

I couldn't help gasping in recognition again and penciling in the margin, like Woody Allen's "Whore of Mensa," "Yes, very true." You see? *Wisdom* is of such a multitasking, infinitely varied scope that I think few men could tolerate it, or even maintain consciousness through it. But they remain ignorant at their peril!

All of that said, even under my inspiring leadership, it is unlikely the targeted demographic of women will ever engage in Bloomsday-like readings of *Wisdom*, as is done with Joyce's *Ulysses*. (Groused a girlfriend to whom I was manically recommending it: "Why should I bother? Every day of menopause *already* feels like you're reading a 600-page book.") So, for the bloated and tired, let me give you the *CliffsNotes*.

Today women between the ages of 44 and 65 are the largest demographic group. So it's no surprise that Northrup considers menopause a major cultural event. Without going into the sometimes arduous detail other feminist texts do (the rising or falling number of women in government, the social architecture of food-sharing collectives), Northrup suggests this gigantic demographic transition will change society—somehow—for the better. All well and good, no arguments there, but now here comes the juicy core of *Wisdom*:

A woman once told me that when her mother was approaching the age of menopause, her father sat the whole family down and said, "Kids, your mother may be going through some changes now, and I want you to be prepared. Your Uncle Ralph told me that when your Aunt Carol went through the change, she threw a leg of lamb right out the window!"

Although this story fits beautifully into the stereotype of the "crazy" menopausal woman, it should not be overlooked that throwing the leg of lamb out the window may have been Aunt Carol's outward expression of the process going on within her soul: the reclaiming of self. Perhaps it was her way of saying how tired she was of waiting on her family, of signaling to them that she was past the cook/chauffeur/dishwasher stage of life. For many women, if not most, part of this reclamation process includes getting in touch with anger and, perhaps, blowing up at loved ones for the first time. Woo-woo! Duck, Uncle Ralph! Go, Aunt Carol!

In short, never mind the wavy-graph technicalities of all those estrogen/progesterone/FSH fluctuations. Opines the doctor: I think it's useful to get your hormone levels tested. But it's far more useful to tune in to how you're feeling than to focus on a lab test, which gives, after all, just a single snapshot of an ever-changing process.

What the phrase *wisdom of menopause* stands for, in the end, is that, as the female body's egg-producing abilities and levels of estrogen and other reproductive hormones begin to wane, so does the hormonal cloud of our nurturing instincts. During this huge biological shift, our brain, temperament, and behaviors will begin to change—as then must, alarmingly, our relationships. As one Northrup chapter title tells it, "Menopause Puts Your Life Under a Microscope," and the message, painful as it is, is: "Grow … or die."

IT'S INTRIGUING TO ponder this suggested reversal of what has traditionally been thought to be the woman's hormonal cloud. A sudden influx of hormones is not what causes 50-year-old Aunt Carol to throw the leg of lamb out the window. Improperly balanced hormones were probably the culprit. Fertility's amped-up reproductive hormones helped Aunt Carol 30 years ago to begin her mysterious automatic weekly ritual of roasting lamb just so and laying out 12 settings of silverware with an OCD-like attention to detail while cheerfully washing and folding and ironing the family laundry. No normal person would do that—look at the rest of the family: they are reading the paper and lazing about like rational, sensible people. And now that Aunt Carol's hormonal cloud is finally wearing off, it's not a tragedy, or an abnormality, or her going crazy—it just means she can rejoin the rest of the human race: she can be the same selfish, non-nurturing, non-bonding type of person everyone else is. (And so what if get-well casseroles won't get baked, PTAs will collapse, and in-laws will go for decades without being sent a single greeting card? Paging Aunt Carol! The *old* Aunt Carol!)

One could further argue that all of these menopausal women, in fact, represent a major evolutionary shift. Owing to women's greatly lengthened lifespan (from about 40 in 1900 to 80 in 2000 in the U.S.), even the notion of what a woman's so-called normal state is can be questioned: Northrup notes that before this time in history, most women never reached menopause—they died before it could arrive. If, in an 80-year life span, a female is fertile for about 25 years (let's call it ages 15 to 40), it is not menopause that triggers the mind-altering and hormone-altering variation; the hormonal "disturbance" is actually *fertility*. Fertility is The Change. It is during fertility that a female loses herself, and enters that cloud overly rich in estrogen. And of course, simply chronologically speaking, over the whole span of her life, the self-abnegation that fertility induces is not the norm— the more standard state of selfishness is.

WHICH IS TO say, if it comes at the right time, menopause *is* wisdom. For Northrup—whose own passage through menopause included a traumatic divorce, a narrative she relates with regret, but little apology—this seemed to be so. Menopause's liberating narrative dovetails elegantly with a typical Baby Boomer female's biological and chronological clock. When a woman gets married in her 20s, has children in her late 20s or early 30s, and begins to detach in her 40s, look where her nuclear family is by the time she reaches her menopausal wanderlust-filled 50s: her grown-up (say 18-year-old) children are leaving the nest; her perhaps slightly older (say 60-ish) husband is transitioning into gardening and fishing; her aged parents have conveniently died (let's say back—and wouldn't it be lovely?—when they slipped and injured a hip at, oh, 78).

Compare that time line, however, with the clock of my own generation of late-Boomer/Gen X women. Putting our careers and our Selves first, we adventured and traveled in our 20s, settled down and got married in our 30s, got pregnant (or tried to—fertility problems being the first surprising biological wall we hit) in our late 30s or even early 40s ... and now what scenario will we face when we hit menopause?

In my case, when it arrived at 49, perimenopause was terrifying, and like nothing I had ever before physically experienced. It was not just the hot flashes, it was the mood swings, although the phrase *mood swings* sounds far too cartoon-like and teen-girlish. I would describe it as the sudden onset of a crippling, unreasoning gloom. It is like resting one's hand on the familiar wall of one's day—helping kids with homework, some grocery shopping, hurtling along on a favorite freeway, listening to Miles Davis—and then feeling the hand suddenly push through the wall, through foam spongy as the flesh of a drowned corpse, into … nothingness.

You experience anxiety at the notion of being face-to-face with your loved ones, because they will immediately read from your dull eyes that which you can no longer hide—that you don't love them, never will again. (And note that I had already divorced my husband of several decades and had run off with my demon gypsy lover … Now I felt repulsion upon hearing the squeaky wheels of the recycling bin he was dutifully rolling out to the curb.) At one time, the sweet smell of your baby's head was your whole world; now you can feel the clanging chime of her 10-year-old voice, note by note, draining your will to live. Where once you coordinated 70 volunteers and thousands of dollars of fund-raising with four- and fivefold Excel spreadsheets at your kids' school, now the mere thought of trying to figure out how to pay the United Visa bill online makes you so depressed, you can't get out of bed. Your chemistry has changed—*and that is no small thing.*

Even more unsettling is how, at night, the depression and anxiety are so much stronger and more intense than the minor quotidian irritants that seem to be tipping you off into hopelessness (the overflowing laundry basket, the $530 car-repair bill, the fact that the scale says you're up—what is it?—eight pounds). The other night, I was awake at 3:24 a.m. as usual (melatonin, Tylenol PM, Ambien, forget it—I could take them all at once, paired with a bottle of wine, and still drive an 18-wheeler). As I lay in the darkness, all at once, the name *Brian Hong* surfaced in my consciousness and I experienced not a passing wave of despair, but despair simply moving in as a cold, straight tide.

I have no idea who Brian Hong is—I was filled with gloom simply because of the name. Perhaps there is, in fact, a lone forgotten yellow Post-it, somewhere on my roll top desk with its gas bills and Discover-card solicitations and Blue Cross health-insurance forms, that reads BRIAN HONG. Perhaps Brian Hong is the head of a small Asian non-profit who several months ago earnestly if a bit keeningly e-mailed me, citing as a referral the name of a mutual friend, to ask if I would drive an hour down to San Pedro to give a free speech at a fund-raising benefit for a flailing youth center for depressed gay minority teens at 10 a.m. three months from now on a cloudy Wednesday.

On the one hand, as a long-time veteran of the non-profit world, I can no longer afford to humor the endless requests to do everything for free, particularly because no one treats you worse than the penniless. On the other hand, though, for me to categorically say no seems like a kick in the teeth to all the kids in the world who are already down; the result of this discomfiting indecision being that I NEVER REPLIED TO BRIAN HONG AT ALL, and so now, like that forgotten spongy corpse, he has come after me in the middle of the night to gently (because that is Brian Hong's passive-aggressive way) but persistently (because that is also Brian Hong's passive-aggressive way) haunt me. Brian Hong! Brian Hong! Brian Hong!

AND OF COURSE, you can only expect it to get worse. I am a member of the "sandwich" generation, that group that must simultaneously care for elderly parents and support children. Never mind that I have lost the dreamlike 40-ish haze I was in during nursing and babyhood and toddlerhood, when the peach fuzz of my daughters' cheeks made for a heady narcotic, when my heart thrilled at all their colorful pieces of kinder art, when I honestly enjoyed—oh the novelty, for someone who had pursued abstract subjects in college and graduate school for 10 years!— baking birthday cakes. Fifty-ish now, when I squat over to pick up their little socks and snip quesadillas into little bowls and yank fine hair out of their brushes, as I have now for the thousandth time, I feel like I'm in a dream, but a very bad, very sour-scented dream. I am fast losing patience with the day job of motherhood. Worse yet, I'll be in the full fires of menopause just when my girls are in the full fires of adolescence! (As my good friend, the family therapist Wendy Mogel, observes, in her calm Zen/Torah–like way, "What wonderful insight you'll have into their mood swings.")

Meanwhile, my Shanghai-born father is 90 years old, has Parkinson's, and is in a wheelchair … But that doesn't mean, with his eerily Jack LaLanne–like resting pulse of 38, he isn't frighteningly willful and able. Every day, my dad wheels himself down to the bus, shouting at his Malibu neighbors and at passing Mexican day laborers to help him; three hours later (via a trip that involves several bus transfers and all the shouting for help that comes with), he arrives at the UCLA campus, where he crashes chemistry and neurobiology lectures, wheeling himself to the front row, asking loud questions, disrupting the class, then going to the bathroom, getting stuck in the stall, and ordering Ph.D. students to help him. The bewildered science departments have been calling us, as well as the UCLA campus police, asking us to remove him or at least assign him a caregiver. We have to reply that we *do* have a full-time caregiver, but my father is impatient to get out in the mornings, won't wait, and indeed, just as often, enjoys the sport of evading capture. I myself have chauffeured my father around, but eventually found myself unwilling, when the men's room was five feet away, to continue to (manually) help him urinate on the street.

In light of my father's situation, I have to question some of the clear-seeming lines Northrup draws. As she puts it:

Learn the difference between care and overcare. True care of others, from a place of unconditional love, enhances our health … That's one reason why volunteering and community service feel good and are associated with improved health. Overcare and burnout result from not including ourselves on the list of people who require care … The way to tell the difference between the two is to be aware of how caring for another makes you feel. You must also be 100 percent honest about what you're getting out of excessive care giving.

Pretty easy for you to say! The problem is, "overcare" is the only thing that ensures functioning lives for the many people who depend on the average woman. Sure, I *could* give it up—but the police and neighbors call every single day of the week, *every single day*. Who's going to do the caring if I don't overcare?

How often do I feel, midlife, as though I am in a strange *Island of Doctor Moreau*–like science experiment? My preteen daughters are flashing more and more midriff as they cavort to the (PG or R? If I could only make out the LYRICS!) gangsta rap of Radio Disney. My ridiculously old father is a giant baby who wheels his own crib into traffic, pees into a Starbucks cup, and still wields, intact, his own power of attorney. As I grow ever more sullen about it all, I feel I should be living alone in a perimenopausal cave.

So, who will supply all the care giving when a whole sandwich generation of 50-ish women checks out? Maybe it will be men: related and hired men. I think of a phalanx of us standing recently in my father's dining room in Malibu, trying to figure out a schedule for his care—or at the very least, for his capture. (From their homes in Northern California, my brother and sister provide all the financial and emotional support to all the caregivers, which is considerable.) In the room at that moment were my Chinese stepmother (74), myself (49), Filipino Nurse No. 1 (female, 60), Filipino Nurse No. 2 (female, 59), and Filipino Nurse No. 3 (male, 41). Who of us were going to take care of my dad? Since all of the women in the room knew all too well the difference between care and overcare, essentially everyone has now quit except for the 41-year-old male, who alone has the strength to heft my dad's wheelchair in traffic, needs the money to support his own family of six, and is paid accordingly (which is to say well, far better than many young college graduates I know). I think also, thank heaven, of my girls' 50-something father, he who holds up the other end of the 50/50 custody balance beam. He is unfailingly calm and patient, buys them fashionable new jeans and tennies, braids their hair, punches new holes in their pink belts, takes them camping, cooks them baked beans, and butters their corn on the cob. By a natural chronology that doesn't imprison *him* in this *Island of Doctor Moreau*–like time line—given that he would not have dreamed of wanting to do all this as a touring musician of 25—my ex, I think, became a father at just the right stage, which is to say older. At his age, my girls have such a wonderfully nurturing father, he might as well be a mother.

I FINALLY WENT FOR some estrogen replacement to the woman who would turn out to be my fabulous new gynecologist, Valerie—who is *not* in my Anthem Blue Cross PPO plan, but whom my demon lover insisted I go to anyway because that was our lesbian neighbors' recommendation.

With kind blue eyes and a comfortingly patterned knit cardigan, exuding an air that you might expect from a Scandinavian maiden aunt, Valerie gently interviewed me—while continually handing me tissues—as I sat on the archetypal metal table in my own paper gown, weeping for what seemed like an hour. And I must tell you—as a middle-aged woman who labors mightily every day to wear the mask of being sane, admitting to experiencing only the narrowest spectrum of emotions, from good-humored cheer to only the lightest irritation, a mood soothed easily with a good chuckle thanks to NPR—that it is beyond delicious to ramble aloud about the infinite varieties, colors, and shades of one's depressions and to discuss, ad nauseam, a month's worth of various panic attacks (going heavy to light, light to heavy). Valerie, listening quietly, wrote down the dates of my periods on a tablet, lending my ravings a reassuring scientific structure, then she gave me one of the most deeply comforting speeches I have ever heard (who from central casting would you get to do it? Streep? Mirren? Lansbury?):

"Sandra," she said, "I have this theory. Let me see if I can describe it for you. I think some girls are paper-plate girls, and some are Chinets. Paper plates collapse even if they have nothing on them; Chinets can take a lot heaped on them and never break. Yes, right now things feel very unstable, and you're having an emotional response to what is a purely physiological phenomenon. But I think, at heart"—and here she leaned forward—"you're a Chinet girl. What we'd like to do now is take some of the stressors off your plate, while at the same time temporarily strengthening its foundation." And with that, she gently smeared the tiniest dot of clear estrogen gel on the inside of my wrist, and even though she said it would take a few weeks to take effect, I *instantly* felt high!

In conclusion gentle reader, here are some handy tips, from women who have survived The Change. (These come after the project of draining your parents' savings so Medicare can pay Filipino male orderlies to do everything.)

The first is a fantastically freeing gambit called "Now That I'm 50." As my friend Denise puts it, "Now that I'm 50, I don't visit my fighting in-laws in Cleveland anymore. My husband can go off and see them if he wants to, but I've been doing it for 20 years, and you know what? Never again." (Beat.) "I'm 50!"

Another is one of my own invention that I call "Stuff It, Barbara Ehrenreich." For years, I was afraid to hire domestic help, because Barbara Ehrenreich wrote in *Nickel and Dimed* that to have a Third World woman scrub your toilets is to oppress a fellow sister. But now that I can afford it, and I've come out of denial over the fact that to have a house cleaned professionally is unbelievably fantastic, once every three weeks, I bring in Marta—whom I refer to sometimes as Marta, and sometimes, baldly, as "the maid"—and when I do so, I silently flip Barbara Ehrenreich the finger. I'm (just about) 50!

A third, related, survival tip is to have no shame. The middle-aged women I know, clawing their way one day at a time through this passage, have no rules—they glue themselves together with absolutely anything they can get their hands on. They do estrogen cream, progesterone biocompounds, vaginal salves, coffee in the morning, big sandwiches at lunch. They drink water all day, they work out twice a week, hard, with personal trainers. They take Xanax to get over the dread of seeing their personal trainers, they take Valium to settle themselves before the first Chardonnay of happy hour. They may do with just a half a line of coke before a very small martini, while knitting and doing some crosswords. If there are cigarettes and skin dryness, there are also collagen and Botox, and the exhilaration of flaming an ex on Facebook. And finally, as another woman friend of mine counseled with perfect sincerity and cheer: "Just gain the 25 pounds. I really think I would not have survived menopause—AND the death of my mother—without having gained these 25 pounds."

Sure, we're supposed to take calcium pills to avoid brittle bones and hip injuries at 90, but who worries about living long when we're just trying to get through the day? In the end, the *real* wisdom of menopause may be in questioning how fun or even sane this chore wheel called modern life actually is. And if what works is black-cohosh tea with a vodka chaser, and an overturned Greek chthonic head as a chocolate-fondue fountain, then bottoms up! Avast, ye vampires and werewolves and pirates! *Arrrr!* ■

Menopause

Irregular period
Hot flashes
Mood changes
Sore breast
Chills
Insomnia
Night sweats
Weight gain/low metabolism

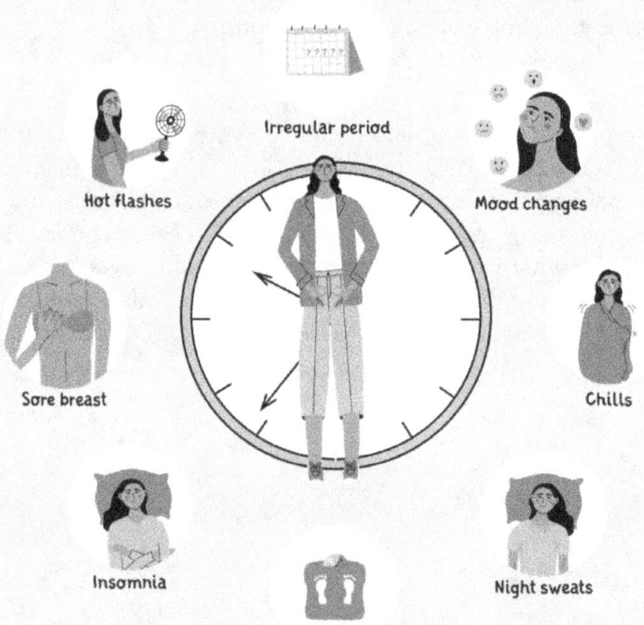

PART 7
PUBLIC FIGURES SPEAK UP!

Wanda Sykes, Comedian & actor

"There's no way in the world men would put up with hot flashes! I think if a man had two hot flashes, they would blow the sun up. You'd go out, they'd got the missile pointed at the sun."

Oprah Winfrey, TV host & producer

My body sent me its first wake-up call more than a year ago, on an evening I'll never forget. One night last June, I—someone who has had every heart test known to womankind and has been repeatedly reassured that I have no blockages—awoke with my heart palpitating so intensely that it felt like it was going to beat right out of my chest. Pound! Pound! Pound! For the first time in my life, I thought I was about to die.

A doctor's visit confirmed what I'd already been told: I don't have heart disease. Over the next six months, my attempts to figure out what I did have led me to four more doctors—and not one could explain the palpitations. Then one morning when I was out running, I mentioned the palpitations to my trainer, Bob Greene.

"I think it's the big M," he said.

"The big M what?" I shot back.

"I think it's menopause," he said.

I stopped and stared at him. "Of course it's not menopause!" I said. "I'm still having my periods. Regular as rain!"

Like nearly every other woman in America, I believed that menopause would hit when my periods ended—that I'd suddenly wake up one day during my fifties in a fit of hot flashing. Yet over the next few days, Bob's words stayed with me: Could he be right? Of the five doctors I'd visited, two were female. Neither had asked whether I, then age 47, might be nearing one of the major markers of a woman's life. I finally put the question directly to my fifth doctor, a heart specialist: Could I be entering menopause? "Well, if it's menopause, ma'am," he said, chuckling, "you're definitely in the wrong place! I don't know a thing about that."

What happened next can only be called a miracle. A few days later, I was walking around the Harpo offices when I noticed a book called *The Wisdom of Menopause*. I opened it right to page 456, where I saw a subtitle that seemed to shout directly at me: "Palpitations: Your Heart's Wake-Up Call." I spotted a woman's story that sounded exactly like my own: "I am a 48-year-old female with no major health problems." Check. "My periods are still fairly regular." Check. "About a month ago...I started experiencing heart irregularities. I felt like my heart was skipping a beat and was going to beat out of my chest!" Double check. Then I saw the line that clarified everything: "There's no question that heart palpitations at menopause are related to changing hormones."

(Before you declare yourself perimenopausal—peri means near or around—hear this: A racing heart could be a symptom of a life-threatening condition, like heart disease. If you experience irregular heart rhythm, please get to a doctor right away.)

Shortly after my revelation, I made a call to the woman who wrote *The Wisdom of Menopause*—Christiane Northrup, M.D., an expert on holistic healing and women's health. Dr. Northrup says that perimenopause begins years before a woman's last period. It can start as early as 35 (yes, 35) and last anywhere from 5 to 13 years. In this country, the average age at which a woman has her final menstrual cycle is 51. And here's a kicker that'll keep you using birth control into your fifties: An entire year must pass after your final period before you can be certain that you've absolutely stopped producing eggs.

Here's what I realized after reading all 498 pages of *The Wisdom of Menopause*: Everything you've always known about taking care of yourself—getting adequate sleep, balancing your diet, drinking water, exercising regularly—comes into sharp focus during this phase. Perimenopause is your body's way of shifting your full attention back onto your well-being. "When you don't take care of your body in your twenties," Northrup says, "you can get away with it. But as you move toward your forties, your body says, 'If you keep this up, I'm gonna make you old—but if you stop now, you'll get a second chance.'"

At Dr. Northrup's suggestion, I cut out what I call the white stuff—high-glycemic-index foods such as potatoes, white rice, refined sugar and bread that throw my insulin level out of whack, cause weight gain, and trigger palpitations. I'd already cut out salt months before, believing that my racing heart might have been a symptom of high blood pressure. After just four days of swearing off the white stuff, my palpitations completely ended.

So many women I've talked to see menopause as an ending—a loss of youth, autonomy and vitality. But I've discovered that the approach of menopause is a knock at the door that can prompt you to finally create the life you've always wanted. This is your moment to reinvent yourself after years of focusing on the needs of everyone else—your mate, your children, your boss. It's your opportunity to get clear about what matters to you, and then to pursue that with all of your energy, time and talent. ∎

Julie Walters, Actor

If you deal with it in a healthy fashion then I think you come out the other side a better person. I've got so much more energy now than I ever had in my early 50s before the menopause.

Kim Cattrall, Actor

I see menopause as the start of the next fabulous phase of life as a woman. Now is a time to tune in to our bodies and embrace this new chapter. If anything, I feel more myself and love my body more now, at 58 years old, than ever before.

Amanda Redman, Actor

How hideous for women of our mothers generation, because - while me and my girlfriends will talk about everything under the sun, including the menopause - it was something they didn't discuss. They must have felt so lonely and embarrassed all the time. For me, it's tailing off now. But I can still suddenly go that awful colour when I'm talking to somebody and sweat beads will break out on my upper lip. You're acutely aware of it, even if they're not. But the more open we are about it, the less of a taboo it will become.

Karen Barber, Former ice dancer and Dancing on Ice judge

The annoying thing is that nobody talks about the menopause. Why is that? It happens to literally every woman in the world, and yet we're all embarrassed about it.

Whoopi Goldberg, Actor

All of a sudden I don't mind saying to people, 'You know what? Get out of my life. You're not right for me.' It's wonderful and liberating.

Florence King, Author

"A woman must wait for her ovaries to die before she can get her rightful personality back. Post-menstrual is the same as pre-menstrual; I am once again what I was before the age of twelve: a female human being who knows that a month has thirty days, not twenty-five, and who can spend every one of them free of the shackles of that defect of body and mind known as femininity."

Jennifer Grey, Actor

"I believe whole-heartedly that age is a mindset. Biological age is what it is, but I truly believe it's more about how you feel—how you feel in your body and how you feel about your body."

Caroline Carr, Author

"The very best way that you can help yourself is to develop and sustain a positive attitude. The way you think and feel about everything will make all the difference to your experience."

Roseanne Barr, Actor and comedian

"I'm enjoying my life, post-menopause, so much. It's just so great to grow into yourself, and not be bothered with all that tyranny of biology."

Sigourney Weaver, Actor

"When you're young, there's so much now that you can't take it in. It's pouring over you like a waterfall. When you're older, it's less intense, but you're able to reach out and drink it. I love being older."

Margaret Atwood, author

"Menopause. A pause while you reconsider men."

Joan Rivers, Comedian

"A study says owning a dog makes you 10 years younger. My first thought was to rescue two more, but I don't want to go through menopause again."

Michelle Obama, Author

"The changes, the highs and lows, and the hormonal shifts, there is power in that. But we were taught to be ashamed of it and to not even seek to understand it or explore it for our own edification, let alone to help the next generation."

Hillary Clinton, Politician

"Women are always being tested … but ultimately, each of us has to define who we are individually and then do the very best job we can to grow into it."

Diane Keaton, Actor

"If I wanted to be prettier, fillers, Botox and a neck lift might help — but I think I'm past all that. My feelings come out in my face and show who I am inside in ways that words can't express. In fact, I'm confused by what 'authentic' is; am I less authentic because I wear 'eccentric' clothes and hats? No. I look at my contemporaries who have had 'good work' done; are they less authentic? No! And neither are the women who've had procedures that went awry."

Suzanne Somers, Actor

"One thing I love about aging—and I do love aging—I've got a wisdom that no young person can buy. You earn it."

Sharon Stone, Actor

"You have to sit down and take a good look at yourself, particularly as you grow older and your face changes. People are afraid of changing; that they're losing something. They don't understand that they are also gaining something."

Gwyneth Paltrow, Actor

"I think menopause gets a really bad rap and needs a bit of a rebranding. I don't think we have in our society a great example of an aspirational menopausal woman."

Cindy Crawford, Model and TV personality

"You start out happy that you have no hips or boobs. All of a sudden you get them, and it feels sloppy. Then just when you start liking them, they start drooping."

Lauren Klarfeld, Author

"As our body journeys through life, and life journeys on our body…. life will leave marks on us too. From the creases of our wrinkles to the birthmarks on our bodies to the tattoos we decide to place."

Victoria Moran, Author

"Growing into your future with health and grace and beauty doesn't have to take all your time. It rather requires a dedication to caring for yourself as if you were rare and precious, which you are, and regarding all life around you as equally so, which it is."

Linda Robinson, Author

"I have to start loving what comes next and stop hating it. I won't be a part of it."

Bonnie Marcus, Author

"Be proud of how you show up every day, feeling comfortable in your own skin, being your magnificent you."

Marianne Williamson, Spiritual teacher and author

"One of the ideas we must agree on and continue to forge with individual and collective vigor is that a woman's life goes uphill at forty."

Ashton Applewhite, Author

"Fear of dying is human. Fear of aging is cultural."

Sandra Tsing Loh, Author, professor, actor

"In the end, the real wisdom of menopause may be in questioning how fun or even sane this chore wheel called modern life actually is."

Trisha Posner, Author

"Our mothers were largely silent about what happened to them as they passed through this midlife change. But a new generation of women has already started to break the wall of silence."

Lisa Jey Davis, Author

"You can do this—this thing, where your body will cease to produce hormones and your skin, hair, muscles and bones … basically every part of you will notice, go into withdrawals, and stage a coup. Be prepared for this mentally, and you'll own this 'thing.'"

Kate Winslet, Actor

"Confidence comes with age, and looking beautiful comes from the confidence someone has in themselves."

Jennifer Aniston, Actor

"I think our bodies are beautiful, and I think celebrating them and being comfortable in them—no matter what age you are—is important. There shouldn't be any kind of shame or discomfort around it."

Heidi Klum, TV personality, model

"I don't think of getting older as looking better or worse; it's just different. You change, and that's okay."

Cynthia Nixon, Actor

"The freedom that comes from no longer being fertile is huge."

Jennifer Lopez, Actor

"When I turned 40, I was like, huh. I accept myself more now. It was much more comforting."

Drew Barrymore, Actor & TV host

"Gravity and wrinkles are fine with me. They're a small price to pay for the new wisdom inside my head and my heart."

Eliza W. Farnham, 19th century novelist, feminist

"And for her true womanhood arrived here there is no growing old. Age refines and enriches, warms and illuminates, expands and exalts her. She is more and more Woman through it; not less and less. The noble life that has let her hither is her grand cosmetic. Her intellect, loosed from the golden bonds of corporeal Maternity, rises to the grasp of higher truths."

Lulu Hunt Peters, M.D.

One should remember that the menopause is a normal and natural process, and it should not be dreaded. Realizing that the condition is a natural occurrence which all women experience—if they live long enough—and a philosophical calm acceptance of this fact, will help lessen the nervous symptoms." .

Cameron Diaz, Actor

"My belief is that it's a privilege to get older. Not everybody gets to get older."

Emma Thompson, Actor

"The trick is to age honestly and gracefully and make it look great so that everyone looks forward to it."

Terri Hanson, Actor

"For many women who have been caring for and putting others first, midlife is the time when there's finally space to start thinking about you. You may feel compelled to make room for you, to live with greater purpose, or to answer the call to do something big in the world. It's during this time that we can begin to define what legacy we want to leave."

Gertrude Stein, Author

"We are always the same age inside."

Morgan Harper Nichols, Artist

"One day you will look back and realize all along you were blooming."

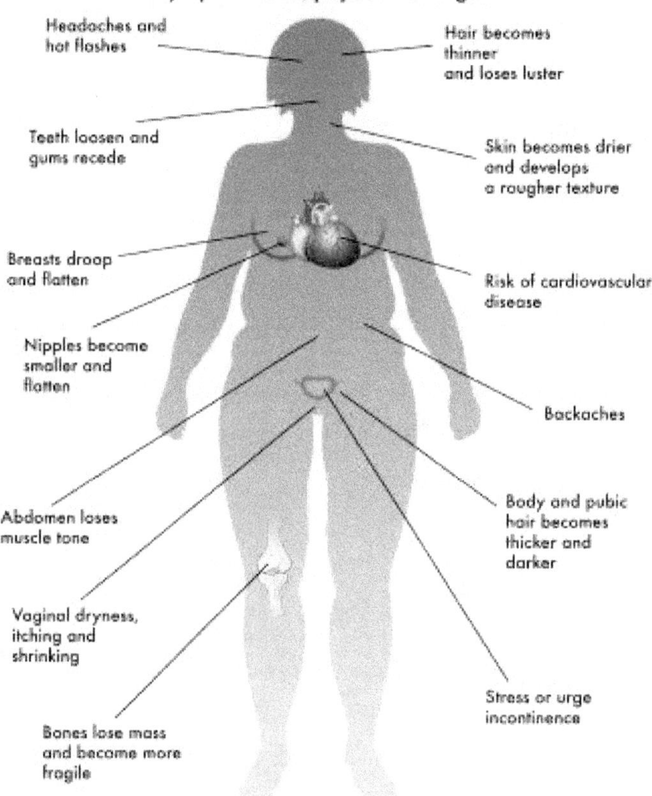

Menopause
Symptoms and physical changes
Headaches and hot flashes
Hair becomes thinner and loses luster
Teeth loosen and gums recede
Skin becomes drier and develops a rougher texture
Breasts droop and flatten
Risk of cardiovascular disease
Nipples become smaller and flatten
Backaches
Abdomen loses muscle tone
Body and pubic hair becomes thicker and darker
Vaginal dryness, itching and shrinking
Stress or urge incontinence
Bones lose mass and become more fragile

PART 8
ONLINE CHATS & FORUMS

I absolutely love the candid responses on the online forums, I think it's often easier to express difficult things honestly in this setting. Here are online chat responses to the question:

Women who have gone through menopause, what was it like for you?

blue-butterfly

I'm 70, and I would say that going through menopause and what's it's like afterwards are pretty much unique to each woman, depending on the hormonal balance you have become accustomed to, and your own one-of-a-kind nature. I was always a highly anxious, fearful person, and have felt calmer and more at peace in the years since. Also, I always, since puberty, had huge hormonal swings with accompanying physical symptoms and mood swings, and it is a great relief to have moved beyond all that. My menopause itself stretched out over years, and was complicated by large fibroids which triggered some frighteningly profuse incidents of blood loss. However, luckily fibroids tend to shrink and go away after menopause. Hot flashes were especially troubling in summer when they seriously interfered with sleep. However, I have friends who had more balanced hormonal systems, and hardly noticed menopause going on except that their periods became lighter and less frequent and eventually stopped. I still get the occasional hot flash even now. But I really do feel so much more in harmony with myself and the world than I ever did as a young woman. I am not sure whether to see that as a result of massive amounts of inner work I have done, or getting past menopause, or both. Probably both and more. But it surely does feel great. Old age is by far my favourite stage of life. ◾

knowonuno

Hi :) I'm 51 and have been on HRT now for about a year. The first symptoms I noticed related to my 12 year depression and anxiety, were mainly horrendous mood swings and exacerbated anxiety. I've always suffered from PMS but this was something else! My poor husband. Nothing was right, I complained and nitpicked at everything, couldn't sleep as my mind was racing about everything bad that had, and could possibly happen in my life, and this was probably for 3 weeks out of the 4. This was the worst thing for me.

Another symptom I had was the hot flushes. I was on Clomid for fertility years ago and had the same feeling then. It's like a weird tingling in my stomach that radiates outwards with heat.. not like being hot from an external source, it's a very odd feeling.

I went to the doc who prescribed Femoston - estradiol and dydrogesterone. They have helped with the mood swings but I'm still getting the tingly heat thing at night sometimes, so at my review in May It may need to be changed. For me, the psychological aspect has been hard. I have 3 children in their 20s and had my tubes tied years ago, but the fact that Mother Nature is now pointing her finger and saying in effect 'you're done!' is hard for me and probably for a lot of women. It's also the fact that we're 'tipping over the edge' into the next phase of life. I'm sure it's difficult for men too, getting older, but women have the definite physical phases that define the stages of life. I admit I've cried about it at times.

I would say if you have unpleasant symptoms then see a doctor. If you have people around you that you can talk to, then talk to them. It's a difficult time of life and the more support you can have, the better. ◾

P_Grammicus

My periods stopped. Like a tap being turned off. It was a complete shock. I tended to have little to no pre-menstrual symptoms and relatively irregular periods, so it took a couple of months for the shoe to drop.

I had little to no psychological symptoms, thank goodness, and it did not affect my mood. I noticed a definite change in my skin about a year after my periods stopped. I've also noticed, several years in, that those skin changes have also affected my labia and vagina. I've always used high quality lube, but intercourse became quite painful. Topical hormonal creams have fixed 99% of those issues, however. My sex drive has probably decreased slightly, though it's still pretty healthy, and my sexual response is excellent, I don't think it changed in a major way at all.
I have a health condition that often comes with night sweats and spontaneous overheating, so the hot flashes likely got mixed in with those. I've always found them very annoying, but after about five years those have decreased a great deal, both in frequency and intensity.
Overall, I was very lucky, especially considering my health. I will add that, other than the skin changes, I was looking forward to menopause and didn't have any issue at all with it from an emotional point of view. I'm very happy to be a crone. ■

japaneseknotweed

SLEEP DEPRIVATION! -- and resultant aphasia!
One of the biggest things that seems to go mostly unnoticed is that all of the heavy bleeding, the hot flashes, the rampaging anxiety, the cramps, whatEVer, makes you sleep like crap.
I didn't get more than 90 minutes of sleep at a time for six months, partly from major hot flashes every forty minutes, partly from chronic pain from a lovely thing called Frozen Shoulder Syndrome.
The CIA uses this as a torture technique. So does Game of Thrones. It's a personality-breakdown method.
Without *deep* sleep, your brain doesn't recharge. Without *uninterrupted* sleep, you can't go deep.

About a month into the other symptoms, I started losing nouns. First one every few hours, then one every paragraph, then one every sentence. I seriously thought I had a brain tumor. I could see the pencil, I could describe the pencil ("long yellow grey inside you write with..." but I couldn't *say* "pencil". Or "dog" or "refrigerator" or the names of dozens of people I've known for years.

It wasn't until a year *after* that a doctor friend put it together. I mentioned a time in my life when I just couldn't form a fluid sentence without stumbling over disappearing words, and she said "Were they nouns? " -- and I said "YES!!!" -- and she said "Were you sleep deprived?" and I said "YES!!!" and she shrugged and said "There you go."

This is SO untalked about, and it has such profound effects. Same with people with injuries or chronic pain issues.

So many of the other symptoms line up with sleep deprivation once you know to look. ■

JoleneAL

Don't hate me!

But my monthly stopped. When I went to the doctor he said - When did your mother and grandmother go through the change? So, I went and found out. It was at the same age I was.

And that was it.

No hot flashes. No nothing.

Just done. ■

Maggiemayday

I started perimenopuase at 47 because I had to take Tamoxifen, an estrogen blocker, for five years after my breast cancer. Finished taking it, and BAM! regular periods again until age 57. Then the periods began to be now and then. Occasional mild hot flashes, some fatigue, definite sleep disruption, and foggy meno-brain. I'd go six months without a period, then have a light one. Took for-freaking-ever to stop. Yes, mild depression, but not sure if it was menopause or health related. Mood swings, yes. Madwoman would be an apt description some days.

Physical changes include drier, snaky skin and lips, and I feel my hair may be thinning slightly. Zero libido most of the time, and we have to use generous amounts of lube for sex to happen at all.

I cannot have HRT because my breast cancer was ER+. ∎

frothulhu

Hello. I'm 29 and am currently post menopausal. I'll preface this by saying that my current experience with menopause is going to be different due to the circumstances behind it.

I have endometriosis and opted to have a bi-lateral salpingo oophrectomy and hysterectomy at the age of 28 to alleviate the symptoms. This of course put me into menopause. I was prepared for it due to having been on chemotherapy for six mo this which also put me into menopause. Due to the chemo I couldn't take hrt aside from progesterone which did nothing to alleviate the hot flash symptoms.

I got the full gamut of bad shit. Mood swings, crying at the drop of a hat, hot flashes, no sex drive at all. I was miserable. My doctor put me on a low dose of testosterone which helped some symptoms like the energy levels and the sex drive but I was angry all the time and my skin was horrible. After the surgery I went hormoneless for a week and spent an entire Sunday crying because I was asked to move back upstairs from the couch. My doctor put me on HRT and things have been relatively okay since. My moods are finally stable and I don't seem to experience depression as easily though my anxiety is worse if I forget to change my patch. My energy levels are eh but I'm not in pain anymore so that's the biggest upside. I currently use the ortho Eve's patch as my hormone replacement as my insurance doesn't cover the HRT my doctor wants me to take. The patch is free so I take that and it works fine. ∎

tinywitch

Dealing with surgical menopause now (apologies in advance for a likely wall of text). I have Stage IV endometriosis and had both ovaries and fallopian tubes removed about 6ish years ago. To put it simply, surgical menopause is a bit different than natural menopause; during natural menopause, hormones typically peter off over the years. Thus, it's a gradual transition. Surgical menopause is immediate and drastic. They removed my ovaries, and BAM--Turbo Menopause at 23.

As far as traditional symptoms, I get monstrous hot flashes. It feels like fingers made of steam start at my throat and fill up my neck and head. I often go and stand in front of the freezer at work. I'm on HRT and that helps a lot.

I had very serious problems with depression and anxiety as a teenager. Like... numerous hospitalizations type of bad. Save for a period of about 3 months post-op (and few and far between day-long episodes), my depression is gone. It's absolutely bizarre and I've never been able to figure out why. My anxiety has gotten better as well. Bodies and brains are weird. It's almost like I morphed into an I-don't-give-a-goddamn-fuck old lady while I was under the knife. This has been absolutely *liberating*.

Forgetfulness has been a serious pain in the ass. It's hard to tell if it's from menopause or from another illness I have called fibromyalgia. Mostly I've been affected by aphasia--the inability to remember words, specifically the names of things. I'll forget the word for cup, for grass, for microwave, etc. Luckily my husband has been great and can typically understand what I'm trying to say. With multiple chronic illnesses it's sometimes hard to tell which symptom is caused by which illness, but I'm willing to bet a lot of it is caused by the surgical menopause.

My frustration tolerance has taken a big hit. It was fairly non-existent before, so this part has been rough. I deal with a lot of weird phobias (they were there way beforehand) so it's made my life a little more difficult. I don't get angry, I get frustrated/overwhelmed. Luckily I'm under the care of a really great psychiatrist and medication has helped.

Keep in mind that a lot of my symptoms are more drastic than typical menopause, but this is mostly what menopause looks like for me as I'm pushing 30. It's really not that bad, especially considering I'm comparing it to what my life was like before with the monster that is endometriosis.

ETA: After reading some of the comments in this thread I realized I didn't even mention my vagina. It's a fucking desert down there. Natural lubrication is a joke at this point. I expected it, but ugh! My husband and I have always made a point to have good-quality lube around since the surgery but there was one time we forgot we were out and it was really late at night. That was a "welp, we are sooo not having sex tonight" moment. It sucks but it's really nothing lube can't fix. Yay, desert vagina. ◼

nikmeone

I'm really thankful you asked this question. It's really helped me to read so many responses from others. I'm 46, started perimenopause around 39? Was really slack about going to the Dr, so it took a few years to get diagnosed. I had horrendous hot flashes, insomnia, fatigue, weight gain, and the worst one was anxiety. I lost all my drive, became a major procrastinator, and honestly felt like there was someone else living in my body. I've been on hrt for 2 years. Within a month, I had a near total transformation. No hot flashes, my drive and energy came rushing back. I felt like me again. I still struggle with very bad anxiety, and it sucks. But some of that may be due to other life stuff over the last few years. I'm starting a course of CBT soon, which I hope will help. At the moment every day is a struggle. ◼

sbsb27

Late 40's started to have night sweats - full soak through your clothing, sheets, pillow night sweats. I was up in the middle of the night just to change clothing. Started HRT and that relieved the hot flashes and sweating - yay! The length of my periods shortened but they were still regular for the next few years. Then my periods became fewer and fewer and ceased entirely by my middle 50's. It seemed time to take me off HRT. I can't speak to depression because I was going through a divorce at the time. It's complicated. It is somewhat of a relief not to deal with menstruation and cramps and bloating anymore. However, it is more difficult to come to orgasm. So enjoy it while you can. ◼

buchliebhaberin

Hot flashes and insomnia are the two worst things I deal with. I can't remember the last time I got a full night's sleep. I also find the "menopause" brain to be annoying. I sometimes have a difficult time recalling names and words. Since I used to take a great deal of pride in remembering names, it is especially galling to now be so forgetful. ■

she-huulk

Another "not me, but..."
My mom went through early menopause so she was just only in her early/mid 40s. My siblings and I were all under the age of 16 I think. My mom was a psychopath. She was so irrational about everything and even the slightest thing would set her off. My dad suffers from mental health issues so my household was pretty fucked for awhile with two insane parents hahah I found out years later that she had to go on SSRI's because it was that bad but then she hated them.....ended up taking hormone replacements and got through the hot flashes etc and now she's must more even keeled. It was definitely hell for both her and the rest of us when it was happening though. ■

OoLaLana

My hormones went *way* out of whack. It was an extremely difficult time for me.
The impact on my job as an executive assistant where I had to be extremely organized and on the ball and paying attention to detail and plan ahead... was excruciating. For over 30 years I'd built a reputation of respect and professionalism with my colleagues... and suddenly I felt like I was losing my mind and couldn't function normally.
Scatterbrained, unfocussed, panicky and extremely uncomfortable with sudden hot flash surges where I'd be removing my jacket and wanting to tear off my clothes... I hated going to work. Each day was unbearable.
My doctor put me on hormone therapy (HT) and I was thrilled. I got my brain back!
Unfortunately a side effect of taking HT was I developed gall stones. (Passing a gall stone while on my knees in the middle of the ER is an unfortunately crystal clear memory that will forever stay with me... but hey, a hip-hip-hooray for my first and only experience with morphine.) I went

off HT, had surgery to remove my gall bladder, and returned to work...
again feeling like I'd lost my mind and couldn't function.

The only thing that got me through was that I'd been planning for the last
10 years to retire at 55... so it was just a matter of months till I could escape
this daily hell and stay home and be somewhere that it didn't matter if I felt
anxious and stupid.

Not a fun time but so relieved and grateful to be on the other side of it.
Life is good. I love my life. ■

CheekyMonkeyMama

I went through early menopause and didn't even know it was happening. I
started peri in my mid thirties, and the doc just thought my periods were
weird (would bleed every two weeks for a week at a time - really dark
colored blood). Anyway, at 40, periods just stopped. My mood stabilized, I
was in heaven - and then the hot flashes started.

I was always the woman who needed a sweater. 90 degrees outside?
Sweater. Beach? Sweater. Now if it's about 72 degrees I feel like I'm dying.
It's definitely worse at night. The house thermostat is set to 70, and I am
literally dripping sweat. If it's humid out, it's even worse.

I was on HRT, but I started to get my period again (or at least bleeding),
again it would be twice a month, and my moods went wacky again. I
decided a few weeks ago, that it wasn't worth it, and stopped the HRT. Hot
flashes are back with a vengeance, but I feel like I'd rather deal with that
then make my family deal with the mood swings.

As a side note: At the same time my periods stopped, the period bowel
movements stopped, then bowel movements stopped all together. Turns
out my colon died, and had to be removed. Trying to separate what
complications I'm having because of that, and what problems are being
caused by menopause has been incredibly difficult. ■

notlikeme

I am 47, and I am hitting the last part of perimenopause and heading into the real deal for the last 6b months. I had never had a panic attack until about 6 months ago and that really sucked. Hot flashes suck. Not being able to sleep sucks. Not having a period is ok, but kind of weird. I only get them about once every 3-4 months now and that has been kind of good, but also kind of weird because there is still that thought that I might be pregnant. I guess it will take awhile to get used to that.
I just feels like sometimes it isn't me anymore, but I really haven't changed that much. that I am actually getting old enough to know that that part of my life that was so important for so long will be gone. ■

mountainulm

I am 60 now and menopause was a breeze. I had a couple of night sweats over several years but that was all, no mood swings....you can ask my Ex SO, lol. I have learned that women on a mostly vegan diet have a way easier menopause with lots less hot flashes and mood swings. Seems to be true for me. ■

probably_bananas

I had a complete hysterectomy at 29. Menopause was pretty horrible for a while, night sweats + insomnia made for dreadful nights. I also had unbearable restless legs, I used to think restless legs were some kind of joke that overly sensitive people complained about but holy shit, they were a nightmare. I finally started taking a low dose of Effexor, then it was upped a little bit when I kept on having hot flashes. So, that helped with my depression also. I've been off the Effexor for 1 year and 3 months and next month I'll be 3 years post hysterectomy. But, I think the biggest change I've noticed is my overall temperature is up all the time, I am generally hot every second. I keep the bedroom so cold at night that I have to cover up the dog sometimes. ■

Im6fut3

I am 45, I had to have emergency surgery just over a year ago due to an ovarian torsion. I had a large cyst on my right ovary, bit my left ovary had a huge cyst that flipped my ovary. The surgeon removed all of my left and 75-80% of my right ovaries. He opted to leave me the small amount of the one in order to not put me on HRT. I went from having very regular easy going periods to holy shit is this for real so heavy I can't leave the house periods. They are irregular to say the least and in the past year I have had three of them last over 30 days! I have mood swings and hot flashes and really hate being a woman lately. And from what I understand this is just the beginning? Ugh. ■

Callmedory

I was on the Pill for 26 years (52 now). When I was 50, the doctor wanted me off the Pill to do a hormone check. Well, guess I went through most of menopause already. I had scattered periods for about a year, some hot flashes, etc. But that was mostly it.
I still get flashes sometimes, but not as much/bad/often as a year ago. I can get *really* hot at night, but I've always done that, since I was little. No idea about mood swings, as I've tried to temper my mood and had other health issues that superseded all of this.
So, likely little help aside from "not all women have horrific menopause experiences." ■

Emptyplates

Going through menopause now. The hot flashes were so bad I wanted to kill everyone then myself pretty much daily. I had to carry towels with me everywhere I went to mop up the flop sweat. I couldn't sleep they were so bad. It felt like I was being burned alive from the inside. I finally went to the doctor and started HRT. No more hot flashes and life is so much better. I had an ablation 9 years ago and haven't had a period in nearly 9 years. So that part is fine. Sex drive is insanely high, thankfully. ■

msjules66

I'm 50 and I've been on estrogen for several years because my thinking became so fuzzy I couldn't keep a calendar and my memory became impaired. Mood swings weren't so much an issue as cognitive function. As soon as my gyno prescribed estrogen gel I felt much better. Recently I've learned that if I skip my estrogen several days in a row I become depressed and inexplicably tearful.

Now insomnia has become unbearable in the last few months. I will say this is the toughest thing I have dealt with so far. I wake up nightly with or without hot flashes and I have to keep the room very cool to sleep. I use a sleep medication many nights or I will become a depressed zombie from lack of sleep. Some days I'm so tired I can't go to the gym in the morning and my day is completely ruined. I don't like to take meds but the benefits outweigh the negatives. I hope this doesn't last for years like they say it does because for me it's been rough. ■

Nibbiecat

I am 55 in menopause for 2 years. I was determined to stay medicine free (if possible), and I have so far been able to do it. To be honest, I had more symptoms/issues the 10 years of peri-menopause. (To the uninitiated, perimenopause is the time prior to the full cessation of menses). I have been on an antidepressant for 20 years and about 3 years ago it became less effective. I had to see a new psychiatrist to address this problem, and we have it pretty well taken care of with some adjustments to diet and the addition of a compounded medicine. My major complaint during perimenopause was the hot flashes. Miserable. I have few of those now, but not nearly as many. I do now have pretty significant insomnia. It is difficult to go to sleep and stay asleep. I keep the bedroom cool (temperature), dark, and limit my interaction with screens (TV, tablet, laptop). I take Somnipure, which is an herbal supplement for sleep (Valerian Root and Melatonin). All these things help and I believe it is a phase which may/may not pass, but I try not to focus on it. Positive attitude is paramount and DON'T feel sorry for yourself!! This is a natural process. Let it process and keep your sense of humor. ■

catmassie

I went through menopause during the last several years, during the same time my family was experiencing a major amount of financial and family stress. So it is really hard to separate out cause and effect regarding emotional states. Minor depression and anxiety have been a constant for me and menopause didn't change that. Besides, it runs in the family. Age 51-52 there was a 2 year time of frequent and very heavy periods, to the point of causing borderline anemia. It was almost impossible to leave the house during those times, so so glad that's over with. That finally tapered off to less frequent periods and now at 54 I'm finally done. Yay! The other day I finally removed that tampon I always carried in my purse, just in case. :-) And I've never had a hot flash, not one. ■

ufdrette

I am 54 and went through menopause without a single symptom. I am not sure how common this is, but I did not have one hot flash. I guess I am just lucky, though I still sort of expect symptoms to suddenly appear, lol ■

Rockgurl1967

I'm beginning menopause right now and I've already had enough. I'm depressed, exhausted and feel awful. I can't feel joy about anything anymore and the week before my period is hell. I feel so low and I have deep bone pain and fatigue. I had a testosterone pellet implanted and am taking bioidentical progesterone but it's no miracle cure. I'm in grad school too so this is really taking a toll on my mental health. I feel like a prisoner to my own hormones. It really is quite intolerable. I'm only 49 and this is just the beginning. Periods are getting more irregular and I can't imagine years more of this. ■

This section of comments answers the online question:
What symptoms have you experienced with menopause?

Comment from: Heather , 45-54

I am 53 years old. Severe perimenopause symptoms started at age 34. I almost died this year from sleep deprivation. I have had awful insomnia since age 48, but this year I went 6 months on average of 10 hours per week of sleep and in June I had 6 hours sleep in 14 days, talk about psychosis! Huge unintentional weight loss. I've used every medication, natural remedy available (herbs/diet changes/acupuncture/cognitive therapy) and hormones of all kinds. Estrogen patch helps a little. Totally debilitated. ∎

Comment from: Mandie Jane , 45-54

My menopause symptoms are heavy bleeding, panic attacks, crippling anxiety, insomnia, brain fog, palpitations, hair thinning, mood swings, massive loss of confidence and depression, all since April! ∎

Comment from: Robyn, 55-64

I am 54 years old. I have been without a period for over a year. I am going through many things with menopause, anxiety, depression, fatigue, hot flashes, cold chills, feelings like electrical shocks, and having no interest in sex. I have dryness, soreness and tenderness in my breasts, irritability, sadness and confusion on what's happening to me. I think I have just about every symptom of menopause. I will be seeing my obstetrician/gynecologist to have my hormones checked. I am going absolutely crazy. I feel like I just don't want to go anywhere.

Comment from: Leslie , 45-54

I think I've had every menopause symptom there is: hot flashes, fatigue, brain fog, muscle loss, digestive issues like constipation and acid reflux, muscle twitching, hot feet and ankles, insomnia and vaginal discharge. My heels and buttocks are sore when I sit and stand long, and I have depression and balance issues. I'm single, so having low libido doesn't bother me as much. I've been to all the doctors. Most say a lot of my symptoms are due to anxiety. All I know is that I feel nuts!∎

Comment from: Renee, 45-54

I have had anxiety begin around age 36 and it has continued to worsen through menopause to where I'm frightened all the time. I'm talking about the fog coming in and I feel it's smothering me. I notice I cry easier. I have had Hashimoto's since age 30. I'm 49 now and also have panic attacks, have to take Ativan to get on an airplane when I used to be able to fly in small planes and the claustrophobia is huge. I have night sweats and hot flashes regularly, I carry a fan. Not to mention weight gain, I can't remember stuff. ■

Comment from: erika1360, 45-54

I have been having so many heart palpitations. I would like to know if anyone has found a way to help ease this during menopause. ■

Comment from: TB, 45-54

I am 51 and my misery with menopause started in my 30s; hot flashes, night sweats, nausea, joint pain, dizziness, heart palpitations, feeling far away, anxiety, digestive problems such as bloating, heartburn and acid reflux, burning tongue, headaches and more. I also have irregular periods and mood swings. Reading others' stories helps a lot. I send good wishes to all. ■

Comment from: Faith , 45-54

I am turning 47 next month. I don't know if I'm going through menopause but I do know my body is changing in the last year. I gained a lot of weight, urinating a lot more and I am always sleepy. I am also growing facial hair. I'm late on my period this month, taken 3 pregnancy tests, and all are saying negative, but no heat flashes. ■

Comment from: Diane, 45-54

I am 46 and still have my periods. I have several symptoms of menopause. Hot flashes have increased my anxiety tenfold. Mood swings are awful. Ugly crying for no reason. Weight gain with no change in diet! Headache, numbness and tingling, fatigue. It's affecting my daily activities! ■

Comment from: Dawn, 45-54

I am in menopause and I'm beginning to feel like I have missed the important part of my life. I'm not an emotional person but I'm beginning to be. I feel lost! ■

Comment from: Angi, 45-54

I would like to know if anyone else entered menopause only to have a random period, like me. I didn't have a period for 2 years and then had one. A normal 5 day period like I never stopped. It's been another 2 years and I haven't had another one. I have noticed something though. Once every couple of months I have some kind of hormone fluctuation. I have discharge that I don't normally have. I find myself sexually turned on and my hot flashes temporarily go away. I entered post-menopause a little early. I am 50 next month. ■

Comment from: ImmaMess, 45-54

I just turned 50 in June and haven't had my period for over a year and 1/2. My biggest complaint and absolute torture with menopause is this strange, acute, non-allergic reaction (caused by hormones apparently) to smells that causes non-stop post-nasal drip to the point that I have to spit and hack it out for hours on end. My nose becomes so inflamed I can't blow it so it pours into my throat. I can't even explain how horrible it's been this past year. Wonder if anyone else experienced it. ■

Comment from: Ronnie, 55-64

My menopause symptoms are hot flushes, constant thoughts of death, palpitations, panic attacks and sore joints, along with many others. ■

Comment from: Lla, 45-54

Menopause has been the most horrifying thing to go through. I feel afraid something bad is going to happen, constant worry, anxiety, depression, crying, and not looking forward to things. I want to feel normal again! ■

Comment from: mk, 45-54

This bleeding is never going to stop and I am waiting for menopause. I'm so scared! Today I am just spotting red mucous-y blood when wiping. I'm just waiting for a flooding to happen anytime. I'm scared to leave my room. Why do I just have random flooding with clots with no warning at all that only last a couple of hours, and then it's back to spotting! In my mind, this can only be cancer. ■

Comment from: Skylamor, 45-54

Let me join the party of menopausal ailments. My menopause symptoms are weird unexplainable anxiety that is very uncomfortable, depression, feeling moody, gas, bloating, constipation, nausea, heartburn, stomach spasms, headaches, backache, heart flutters, frequent and/or burning urination when there's no urinary tract infection (UTI). I don't feel like being intimate with my husband… this change has changed me. Don't feel like myself anymore. ■

Comment from: jolly, 55-64

My menopause symptoms are crippling anxiety and very low mood. ■

Comment from: Younganddone, 35-44

With menopause, I have no sex drive, rage, irritability, loss of interest in most things I enjoyed doing, and I just want to be left alone. I also have random cravings, headaches, and muscle cramps in my legs. ■

Comment from: Leah, 45-54

I'm 50, had hysterectomy at 26 and oophorectomy at 35 and developed hot flashes, nausea, severe panic attacks, acid reflux and anxiety constantly, but my doctor won't test me for menopause. I had weight gain but the nausea, vomiting and bowel issues took care of that. ■

Comment from: Carol, 65-74

I had a total hysterectomy at age 41 years. I have been on hormone replacement therapy (HRT) gel for 27 years after menopause. Twelve months ago I came off HRT, and I have severe nights sweats which wake me often through the night. I sleep on towels. I'm so tired and moody all the time. Daytime is not much better, my clothes are always damp and sticking to me. This has been 12 months of torture. I came off HRT as it was not helping with the sweats. Wonder if I am just being a whinger? ∎

Comment from: DearJane, 45-54

I decided to leave this comment in hopes it may help someone else. I'm 52. I started having menopause symptoms at 48. I haven't had a period in well over a year, and my symptoms have steadily become worse. They include palpitations, terrible headaches/migraines, severe fatigue, aches and pains all over including in my chest, mild numbness, hot flashes, nausea, feeling unbalanced/almost dizzy, severe anxiety including attacks, and more. I even went to the hospital, and all tests are normal. ∎

Comment from: Mari, 45-54

I am going to be 50 years old this year. I've been in perimenopause for 10 years and I think I got all the 36 symptoms of menopause! This time my neck, shoulder and upper back ache and pain, and my right hand and fingers are also hurting and swollen. I experienced different symptoms in the past like IBS 9irritable bowel syndrome), acid reflux, bad migraine, leg cramps, allergies, heavy and longer periods and skipped periods (for 7 months), then having a period just like a normal one and then stopped again. Really, so stressful. ∎

Comment from: Mav, 45-54

I am in my 3rd year of no period. It is a nightmare, symptoms upon symptoms of menopause, some you can't describe. My doctor told me that I will never feel better, I am going on 51. ∎

Comment from: Angie, 45-54

Menopause is causing a dreadful rage in me that's affecting my poor family. ∎

Comment from: Vilma, 55-64

I never experienced hot flashes and night sweats with menopause. I did experience very bad anxiety and panic attacks. The persistence of anxiety made me feel very depressed. I had a range of body sensations that were very scary. My doctor did tests and said it was anxiety related to menopause. I started to have digestive issues as well such as reflux. It was very helpful to see a qualified naturopath and a functional medicine doctor. ■

Comment from: Bluecat, 45-54

I wonder if anyone experienced non-cyclical breast pain with menopause. I have a weird prickling sensation in my right breast. To be on the safe side I have referred to the breast clinic who told me it is perimenopause, but I also need extra x-rays and ultrasounds. I'm so scared. ■

Comment from: Nicole, 45-54

For the past 3 days my legs will not stop twitching. I've been to my neurologist the past week and she did check me and all went well. I went to my obstetrician/gynecologist, had blood work, and she said my estrogen is out of whack from menopause. I also get hot flashes. I'm just worried about the twitching and wonder if this has happened to anyone else. Oh, and I'm 48 years old and I have anxiety too. Thank you. ■

Comment from: Cary , 55-64

My symptoms of menopause are hot flushes, anxiety, muscle twitching, and electric shock sensation in my forehead. ■

Comment from: Josie, 45-54

My menopause symptoms are hot flushes, mood swings, depression and headaches. ■

Comment from: Nessa, 35-44

I started with severe anxiety in 2013. I was 36 at the time. Now I'm 43 and have experienced every menopause symptom from palpitations, anxiety, depression to joint pains. Now I have nausea, dizziness and headaches. Also beating in my ears and heat waves. When will it end! ■

Comment from: Fl0gger, 35-44

My menopause symptoms extremely severe; hot flashes (feels like I'm spontaneously combusting), insomnia, weight gain, memory loss, absolutely no sex drive, and mood swings. I also have Hashimoto's. I am so not me anymore! ∎

Comment from: Bellann, 45-54

I am 47. I have been having menopause symptoms for about three years; hot flashes, insomnia at night, anxiety and panic attacks, acid reflux, mood swings, and especially changes in my cycle including shorter cycles, skipped, and sometimes an extra-long cycle. ∎

Comment from: Jamie, 55-64

I've been in menopause for 3 years, and recently I've been sweating on the face heavily, every 15 minutes or so. I don't know if this is menopausal issue and not something else. ∎

Comment from: Kay, 55-64

I'm 57 years old and had no periods for 4 years. My menopause symptoms are so debilitating; dizziness, worsening migraine, balance issues, and loud noise in ears. I cannot take hormone replacement therapy due to breast cancer in close family members. I have been offered anti-depressants, had brain scan and multiple blood tests which are all completely normal. ∎

Comment from: Just me, 65-74

I had my last period at 40 and been in menopause since. I am now 64 and recently began having flashes. I am also losing my hair I have a quarter of the hair I once had. I am not sure this is normal. ∎

Comment from: Raisin, 55-64

I am currently 56, I stopped having my periods at age 52. For me menopause wasn't that big a deal. Yes, I had hot flashes and night sweats, and an occasional sleepless night. It certainly wasn't as bad as I had imagined it to be in my head. I think if you go into it with the attitude that this is a natural part of the aging process that can help you. I can tell you one thing, I'm much happier without my 'monthly visitor' showing up. ■

Comment from: Roni, 55-64

I am going through menopause, age 52. I have anxiety, depression, hot flashes, bloating and acid reflux. Wonder if anyone else has acid reflex and heartburn (sometimes after eating spicy). It was so bad I went to emergency. In CT scan I was diagnosed with gallbladder stone. I am so worried, don't know what to do. ■

Comment from: Ny2Fl, 35-44

I'm 42. I haven't had my period in the last 3 months. I believe I started having menopausal symptoms in my late 30s. I am waking up drenched in sweat, like I had gone swimming. Then I got pregnant with my 3rd child. All born 7 years apart. All C-sections. I had a tubal ligation during the last. He's now just turned 5. I have suffered through the drenching night sweats, but they aren't everything. Mostly I am very emotional. I cry a lot. I have no energy or motivation. Most days I just wish I would die. ■

Comment from: Tilly, 55-64

I reached menopause at 50. I have had terrible hot flashes now going on 9 years. Also, low libido, urinary tract infections, insomnia, irritability, anxiety, mood swings, weight gain, and now having headaches and nausea in the mornings. I am active, love my coffee in the mornings, wine in the evening. I cut those things out, decreased sugars and spice, and no change in any symptoms. I am using prescription low dose estrogen cream which totally took away urinary tract problems! ■

Comment from: Amber, 45-54

I'm 46 and have had horrible heavy periods to the point I was put on low dose birth control. I was on those for 8 months and stopped due to vaginal dryness and painful cramps, plus it stopped working for the heavy flow. So I started taking yarrow, red raspberry leaf, and slow flow supplements. This has helped me so much. Also red clover helps me with night sweats and vaginal dryness. I now use branded progesterone cream as directed, it helps me feel good, and it's calming. Good luck. ■

Comment from: Kathy , 55-64

I am 55 year old, and a year ago I found out I was menopausal. I feel like I'm losing my mind; hot flashes, mood swings, body aches, etc. My doctor won't put me on hormones because of my heart attack in 2014, so I'm going cold turkey and losing my mind. ■

Comment from: Emily, 45-54

I am 46. I have the regular perimenopause symptoms; hot flashes, memory loss/forgetfulness, mood swings, etc. I had a major migraine last month that lasted for 3 days. Ever since then, I've been feeling off balance. It seems that so many of us are experiencing this, but wonder if anybody has found anything to get rid of it. Please don't tell me, time! I hate that answer.■

Comment from: SP, 45-54

I am 54 year old, I had my last period a year ago but had spotting in intervals of 2 to 3 months. Estradiol is 145 and FSH serum is 22.66. I have severe pain in my right leg below the knee (side of the calf muscle) that spreads on my feet, along with cramps like feeling on the legs, fingertips of my hand, and toes too. I am trying my level best to ignore and keep myself busy but it is irritating me a lot. I am extremely distressed and lethargic. Please share if anyone of you is going through this with menopause and the remedy to overcome it. ■

Comment from: AboutmeNJ , 45-54

I feel horrible, my menopause symptoms are very scary, like I think something bad is going to happen to me. I have dizziness to the extreme that I think I am going to pass out, muscular pain mostly of my neck, left side of my chest and arm which makes me think I am having a heart attack. The hot flashes are a weird feeling, they happen 3 to 4 or more times during the day and they wake me up at night. Lately I been having chills, suddenly teeth chattering. I haven't read of many women having these kinds of symptoms. ■

Comment from: Pink, 45-54

I'm 53 and I think I'm finally going through menopause. It has only been a few months though, but my periods have stopped, and no, I am not pregnant. I get hot flashes at night but the strange thing is, I'm not craving sugar or pop anymore. I have or had a huge sweet tooth eating candy or anything sweet during the day and drink 4 to 5 cans of Pepsi a day. Now I am just craving protein before I go to bed which is all good, hopefully I can lose a few pounds but, wonder if anyone else has experienced these symptoms. ■

Comment from: Anxiety is me, 45-54

I have been in menopause for 4 years but ovulation continues. Now I have ovulation with blood and I am freaking out. My mom had uterine cancer 14 years ago. ■

Comment from: Ali, 45-54

Wonder if anyone else has suffered with recurring nausea from menopause like me. ■

Comment from: Alex, 45-54

I started with hot flushes a year ago creeping up my neck to face, and pumping heart; I thought I was having a heart attack. I was drinking alcohol more around my period as this is how I feel. I am trying St. John's wort, black cohosh and passionflower herbs, also going 2 try kudzu and skullcap as I have an herbal medicine book to try and alleviate all these symptoms of menopause. ■

Comment from: Gloria, 55-64

I learned that there is a such thing as post-menopause. I'm on an herbal that is helping. However I do have anxiety during the day, insomnia, and night sweats at night. I am very sensitive and take natural supplements. Hormone replacement therapy did not work for me. ■

Comment from: Eden, 55-64

Been a long way with menopause ladies, but here we are pushing on. Here I am today feeling awful, my one year since menopause is September. I have had anxiety, for a full year it was like this, then I have had all kinds crazy symptoms, but the anxiety is the worst. I don't know what happens, and wonder if this means I'm about to get a period. Oh my, or this is it until 2 or 4 years till the body adapts! I have no one to talk to about this for tons of reasons, I just turned 56. ■

Comment from: LP, 45-54

I began perimenopause at 48, and now 52. It has gotten so bad, hot flashes all day and night, and restless sleep. I have weight gain, bloating all day and night, mood swings; just feeling like a fat, hot, crazy woman. Menopause is awful for me. ■

Comment from: Lewlew, 45-54

I'm 50 years old now. If I think back 2 years, menopause started with major fatigue to the point walking 200 ft. made me tired. Thyroid was fine. But suddenly due to stress, my symptoms kicked in. I never had hot flashes but fatigue, brain fog, lack of motivation, difficulty reading, joy replaced with apathy and not giving a darn, dizziness, withdrawal from being social engagements, joint aches, insomnia, forgetfulness, insecurity, etc. Not all symptoms all the time but these have changed who I am within the past year. ■

Comment from: Tess , 55-64

I had my last period at 48 years old. The hot flashes started with menopause but weren't as bad as the night sweats that interrupted my sleep. Topical bio-identical progesterone helped with those. Then my vagina dried up, so I started bio-identical vaginal estrogen which helped with that. Emotionally, it's been the worst with depression, and anxiety that does not relent. I also can't stand the smell of my husband nor can I lose the weight I have gained. I am not me anymore. ■

Comment from: Menopause and nausea, 65-74

I am 65 years old and started my menopause 10 years ago. I stopped and started HRT (hormone replacement therapy) 5 months ago. Now I am waking up every day feeling very nauseous. I am so tired as the nausea continues for the rest of the morning. ■

Comment from: Marion , 35-44

I am feeling like a blown up balloon during early stages of menopause and at same time periods come twice in a month, then once the next, wonder if anyone else relates to this. I also have diarrhea and cramping stomach pain all night long. ■

Comment from: Tiredmeni, 45-54

At 49 I am experiencing sporadic hot flashes with menopause... wham, there it goes, all of a sudden and wherever I am, they take over, ugh! Sweat drips from my brow and my face is flushed, and don't let me get started on the night sweats… yep, soaking wet, nightly! Very sexy, not! And then there is the lack of interest in sex, poor hubby. Best part of menopause… no cramps and no bleeding. ■

Comment from: Kslh1210, 55-64

I'm 56 and haven't had a period in 10 years. I've been lucky not having very many hot flashes, no mood swings, and what surprised me is I'm not dry like it says you will be with menopause. I'm not sure why that is, also my sex drive hasn't faded either. ■

Comment from: Needing_Help, 45-54

I'm 47 years old and have been post-menopausal over the last 4 years (going on 5). I'm currently on the highest dose of SottoPelle, wear the Combipatch, receive B-12 injections, and eat a very healthy diet. I have no energy! I was an avid runner and ran marathons and 50 Ks up until 2017 and can barely knock out 3 miles now without feeling like death and needing to recover for a week. What is wrong with me! I'm merely existing at this point in life. I enjoy nothing anymore. This is awful. ■

Comment from: Yoland, 45-54

In July 2019 I was having hot flashes and menopause also made my mood change. I was burning up and sweating like I was working out. Also I haven't had a period. ■

Comment from: Laura, 55-64

I am 58 and I've been having anxiety and panic attacks and depression for the last 6 years. I've been diagnosed with depression but no doctor has told me that these symptoms are part of the menopause. I have hot flushes from time to time. I have seen several doctors but not one of them has mentioned the menopause, instead I was treated for depression. It would have been helpful if they had mentioned the menopause instead of just treating me for depression. ■

Comment from: Kiki, 65-74 Male

My wife, 73 years old, a long time since menopause, has been suffering from excessive sweating in her upper body (head, neck and back) for the past 7 months. She says the sweat is cold, and she wears warm clothing and has the heating on even though it is 31 degrees Celsius outside. At nights she must dry her hair with a hair dryer. She has seen her general physician, an internist, a gynecologist, a neurologist, an endocrinologist, a dermatologist, a psychiatrist and a psychologist. She even spent 3 weeks in a psychiatric ward. ■

Comment from: Sam, 45-54 Female

I'm at a total loss, I've lost my mind, I've lost my sex drive, and I lost my sense of humor with menopause. Some days I just can't cope with life. I was an early menopause lady 0.40 mg ten years on hormone replacement therapy (HRT), and now medication free as the only HRT I could take is now discontinued which leaves me high and dry. ■

Comment from: Yolita, 45-54

I'm 48, almost 49, and I still have terrible periods. Here are my menopause symptoms. I only get one good week symptom free. After that I feel crampy, I feel hot at night and lately my back has hurt me so bad I have to miss work. And these symptoms are ongoing for weeks before my actual cycle starts and the cramps are unbearable. It's really starting to affect my life where I don't go anywhere and I miss work where it didn't affect my life that way before. I need some advice on what steps to take. ■

Comment from: Amber, 45-54

I'm 45 and in perimenopause. I was having heavy flooding periods every month and night sweats starting a week prior to periods. I had dryer skin and curly hair going straight. I tried everything natural to calm the heavy periods, nothing helped so my doctor put me on Microgestin FE 1/20. It's wonderful. Very light spotting for withdrawal bleeding, and night sweats have calmed down. I will stay on this pill until 51 or menopause. ■

Comment from: Tricia , 45-54

My period ended very early, at or around 39 or 40 something years of age. I remember around 9 years ago I was feeling like I was going to lose my mind and didn't know what was wrong with me, it turned out to be anxiety and now I also have panic disorder. So my guess is that I was premenopausal and that's why I had anxiety. I am now 52 and the hot flashes, jitters, nervousness, and fast heart rate have started. My doctor said, 'it is time' meaning to get menopause symptoms. I feel awful! ■

Comment from: Onel, 45-54

I am 52 years old and into my menopause; I haven't had my period in 4 months. I get hot flashes like I'm burning up. I have been getting these clear sticky discharges lately. I wonder what that means! There is no odor to it. ■

Comment from: kkkyystone, 55-64

I am 56, my last period was a few months before my 55th birthday so I am officially in menopause. I had a fairly easy time of it until 53 where I had a year of extremely heavy periods and came down with anemia. They wanted to try an intrauterine device (IUD), I tried acupuncture instead. It worked. I had three regular periods and then they stopped. I still get hot flashes and still struggle with some fatigue. I am still trying to lose the 10 pounds I gained. No more periods is great, but the hot flashes are annoying. ■

Comment from: tracy73, 45-54

With menopause I have burning during sex. ■

Comment from: insanityrus, 55-64

I am a 55 year old female who never had a regular period; I would have one for 3 days for 2 months and then not have one for a year or so. I took fertility drugs and had two children. They said my LSH and FSH levels were backwards. I got pregnant for my third child at 35 without any fertility drugs. I was on Depo-Provera for almost 20 years and stopped it four months ago. They said my FSH levels say I am post-menopausal. Due to the Depo I haven't had a period in almost 20 years. I have had urinary incontinence for the last few years, hot flashes for the past few weeks that last for at least 5 minutes apiece, and a brownish discharge for at least a month. If I am post-menopausal I wonder why all this is happening now, but get no answers. ■

Comment from: Chillyhilly, 55-64

Looks like I'm one of the lucky ones. A few hot flashes a day but they don't really bother me. Maybe I am more emotional than I used to be but on the whole no big deal at all. Gone a year without a period now so I'm guessing that's the menopause done. So if you're worrying about going through it after reading all the horror stories on here please stop as you could have it easy too. ■

Comment from: Alice, 45-54

I reached menopause when I was 43. Slowly I had fallen ill, and I started having hot flashes. They were so bad that I used to break out in a sweat every half hour. I found it really stressful. At last with my friend's suggestion, I started using VieBien menopause support, a natural menopause relief supplement. Really it was magic, it ended all my symptoms. ■

Comment from: soi, 55-64

I am 55 years old and still having heavy bleeding with clots, and fever on those days in the range of 99 to 102. I don't know whether it is normal with menopause. The bleeding is controlled with tranexamic acid 500 mg thrice a day. ■

Comment from: Teresa, 35-44

I began at age 39 with breast cancer, then 13 years later, I got bone cancer. The night-time and daytimes heat flashes because of the menopause are awful. I wake up with wet hair and wet shirt. ■

Comment from: amyplus, 55-64

I am menopausal from 4 years, I had just a few menopausal symptoms so I decided not to take HRT (hormone replacement therapy). However, I actually have problems with dryness and irritation of the vagina which makes sex painful, I guess it is due to the lack of estrogen. I was looking for alternatives to manage this problem and I found this new treatment, it seems to be painless and able to solve this kind of problem, it is called Mona Lisa Touch. ■

Comment from LMP 35-44

I'm 37 and am having weird symptoms that I believe to be menopause. I am frustrated at the lack of straight-forward information. For instance, why are they not doing more in-depth studies of progesterone cream, or bioidentical hormones? If men went through menopause, I'd bet they'd have all this figured out by now.... ■

Comment from: snow_hiker, 45-54

I started "the change" when I turned 40. Bear in mind, I only had spotting during my menses, but also suffered cramping so bad the first day, I was on prescription pain pills to be able to function. Even after the birth of my only child at age 32, I continued to only spot, but no more cramps. I have NOT had any surgery to remove my female parts or tie my tubes, everything is still intact. Once I had started the change, I went through what my doctor called "classic" text book symptoms. These included: night sweats, hot flashes, irregular periods (not every month), mood swings, increase/decrease in libido, weight changes, etc.. My doctor told me that once I quit having my menses for a full 12 months, I would be "completed" through the change. He was right, but I still have the occasional hot flashes. He said that can happen and may or may not continue the rest of my life. HE SAID EVERY WOMAN IS DIFFERENT WHEN IT COMES TO MENOPAUSE, AND THAT EACH ONE WILL EXPERIENCE A COMBINATION OF SYMPTOMS. He also SUGGESTED (mind you)that if I could deal with going through menopause and afterwards WITHOUT HRT (hormone therapy), I would be better off without it. SO I CHOSE NOT TO TAKE IT. Not every doctor would agree with that, but I believe he is right. I am now 53 yrs old, and my bone density is still the same as it was when I had my first mammogram at age 39. I take 1200 mg of Calcium with Vitamin D daily, and also go for a walk 3 to 4 times a week. I still have the occasional hot flash, but I can live with that. Not having my periods anymore is so wonderful! Menopause ROCKS!!! ■

Comment from: Hot mess, 55-64

I had a complete hysterectomy in 2011 with both ovaries removed. I wonder if it is possible to still have hot flashes and menopausal symptoms after 10 years! ■

Comment from: Stressed , 45-54

Since menopause I have all day gas and frequency of bowel movements. ■

Comment from: Tyty, 45-54

I am a 50 year old female in menopause since 2017. I had a 3 day bleed 2 months ago. Endometrial lining was found to be 6 mm. Failed endometrial biopsy on 12/24. CA 125 is negative. CT of abdomen and pelvis negative. Estradiol level is 104 pg/ml. I get uterine cramps daily, and pain after food. My breasts are tender. ■

Comment from: Maria, 45-54

I have not had a period since I was 32 years old, and I'm 52. I am getting hot flashes, feel like I can't be, but it seems like menopause. Not sweating, but major flash. Not sure what's going on. Heart rate was found to be fast this year twice. ■

Comment from: Karen, 55-64

I have come off the pill for 6 months now. I have no period but I feel depressed. Wonder if this is menopause. ■

Comment from: Bobby, 55-64

I'm 56 with periods ending 13 months ago. Menopause is worse than premenopausal stage, the anxiety is bad, and everyday feels like a period, wish it would come on. ■

Comment from: Ljules, 35-44

I am 40. My periods always been just medium flow like clockwork until last year when I had a few heavy ones with clots, but still every 28 days. I bled last month as normal but about a week after had two days spotting. Then the next period was 5 days late. I am due on again this weekend but had spotting for 5 days now; just see it when I wipe, and discharge. I wonder if it is menopause or I need to be worried. ■

Comment from: Andrea, 45-54

I feel the same as another commenter here. I feel as if I've lost myself. I take hormone replacement therapy and anti-depressants, and I feel life is not worth living anymore. I don't what to do. ■

Comment from: SOConfused, 45-54

I am confused on what to do. I am 52, feel great, on the pill and no symptoms of menopause. Really kind of best I've felt in a few years. I went to my doctor the other day for my yearly and she insisted I start talking hormones because I am of age. I had no family history of breast cancer and my mom got after she started hormones. She is all good now, but I'm scared to take, especially when I feel great, don't want to get pregnant and kind of being forced to take! ■

Comment from: Wendy , 55-64

I am 58 years old and had a hysterectomy at 44, and still waiting for menopause. Wondering if I could have the luck of no nasty symptoms... or is it going to hit me soon! ■

Comment from: dori, 45-54

I cry it seems almost always, I for the last 3 years have had what I refer to as "gunk", brown discharge along with bleeding. I can't find any info on it, I now for the last 3 months have had almost constant daily nonstop spotting, to the point I always have to wear a pad. I feel depressed, have suicidal thoughts, I wonder how so many woman before me survived this, my husband although for the most part is patient. I think gets just a frustrated as me. I feel alone, our sex life is almost nonexistent which makes me feel distant from my husband of 29 years, I have tried many things, and the only thing that even remotely helps is menocalm, a natural supplement. I feel like I am losing my identity, I want this to end. ■

Comment from: 45-54 Female

I am almost 52 and have all the symptoms of menopause except my periods come every month like clockwork. They have been like that since I was 13, except for pregnancies. I am beginning to think I will never stop. My mom is 72 and takes low-dose hormones and still has a light period. I'm not sure what to make of that. She has no other symptoms and is the healthiest person I know. I am ready for all this to end. ■

Comment from: Lynn, 45-54

Peri-menopause began in my early 40's when I still had all 4 kids at home. My periods would last 10-14 days and heavy, changing pads and tampons sometimes every hour. Then I would have a week off of them and back again. No Dr. took it seriously, that I felt the bottom was dropping out of my vagina. I didn't want to go on field trips or PTA anything! Now I'm 52 and so very thankful to be menopausal. Hot flashes are temporary and I am sleeping better than when in the peri stage when I was also diagnosed with Graves disease. I thought it was all part of the peri stage until I had palpitations. All good now and my husband is ok with the 20 pound weight gain, even if I hate it and when it cools back off here in AZ, I'll be out walking daily again. Hang in there ladies, we've been through worse! ■

Comment from: gdb, 55-64

I certainly wish I could say that menopause is a breeze. It's been anything but, for me. Severe hot flashes began at age 51. They begin at my feet and go up to my head. I feel faint with each one. I hear people talking in the distance first, and then the flash begins. I have them every second week. I'm 55 now. It is still the same. I can have 20 or thirty a day for 3-4 days every second week. Then I get severe anxiety for the remainder of the week. I have severe insomnia, chronic diarrhea, very tender, achy muscles. I have tried everything from synthetic hormones, bio-identical hormones, diet change, and have read whatever I can get my hands on. No success. Oh ya, I also tried acupuncture. Nothing helps. I can honestly say, it's been the worst four years of my life. ■

Comment from: NULL 35-44

I am only 35 and I had to have a hysterectomy due to an illness and now I am feeling as if I have no energy to do anything. I am always crabby and I can't seem to get interested in having sex at all. I pray that I can get some kind of treatment to help me get through this. I am still too young to feel this worn out. ■

Comment from: Elma, 45-54

I have had issues with heavy and painful periods for many years. In 2012 it was so bad I was having such heavy and never ending periods. A gynecologist put me on megestrol. Overnight my periods disappeared and it was like a miracle. I had some weight gain from it as a side effect. I took it for many years until 2019 my prescription ran out and my primary care physician would not refill. I had a sonogram that showed a thickening in my uterus. I had a biopsy that was negative. Meanwhile no medicines. It has been a nightmare. ■

Comment from: Cheryl, 35-44

I have recently been diagnosed with bowel cancer at the age of 37 so having radiation and chemotherapy followed by an operation. While in they are taking my womb as a precaution. I don't know if radiation is making me infertile, but I'm on the Depo-Provera injection so wonder how I will know if early menopause has kicked in. ■

Comment from: Trish19841, 45-54

I have hot flashes more at night. It starts in the evening. I hope this doesn't go on too long! ■

Comment from: cntrygrl55, 45-54

I Started menopause at 42. I lost 30 pounds within the last 2 years. When I started losing weight I started menopause all over again, after thinking I was done with it 13 years ago! I had night sweats, hot flashes, anxiety, panic attacks, and insomnia. ■

Comment from: sex yuck, 45-54

I am 49. I been getting horrible hot flashes for 4-5 years and hate -- I mean hate sex! My husband does not believe hating sex can be because of menopause. ■

Comment from: Rachel 5, 35-44

I am waking up very occasionally with night heat flashes. I have a burning sensation all over and I have increased weight gain. ■

Comment from: Redspyder, 45-54

I have no children and started the change at 34! I had one long, heavy flow, major cramp period, then DONE. No spotting at all. I just turned 45 and still have hot flashes all of the time. I am very emotional and I have ZERO energy. I can't sleep and have to use the bathroom 20 times a day. I am single and probably will be forever as I have no interest in sex at all. I also feel like my brain is mush and can't remember anything. Oh gee, can't wait for my "golden years!" I already feel like I'm 90! ■

Comment from: 55-64 Female

I am 55. I have had enough of these night sweats and not sleeping. This has been going on for about 18 months. My poor husband! ■

Comment from: had enough, 55-64

I'm 55yrs old and have been having menopause symptoms since I was 45. I started with the heart palpitation in the neck, then the cold chills at night. Now I have the hot flashes on and off all day. They do start at the bottom of my feet and work their way up to my head. I have a new symptom now insomnia. I'm tired at night and go to bed at a reasonable time. I lay there trying to sleep but it doesn't come. My doctor gave me a very low antidepressant to take. I hope this works. ∎

The comments below are an emotional online menopause post & resulting supportive conversation in an online forum on Menopause Matters:

Fed up and so very miserable - Biker Chick

Hi everyone

I haven't been on the forum for a while because of one thing or another. I just needed to vent as I'm sat here in my house by myself crying again. That is all I seem to do these days. I'm so unhappy. There doesn't seem to be a light at the end of the tunnel. I often think everyone would be better off without me. I got made redundant a year ago. I'm currently living on benefits and my dwindling redundancy pay as I have been diagnosed with depression and Post Traumatic Stress as well as going through the menopause and am not in the right head space to look for work. I'm currently on the waiting list with IAPT for therapy. Have previously tried CBT but it wasn't for me. Have also tried hypnotherapy. I am not work-shy, I have worked all my life since I was 18, I'm now 53. My head is so full of negative thoughts all the time. I'm constantly thinking of death. Think is as a result of witnessing my partner having a massive heart attack a couple of years ago, luckily he survived. I have then subsequently lost several close people in my life. I've had an awful couple of years. I can't seem to pull myself round. I think I am going mental to be honest. I just want to shut myself away and not bother with anyone. I have told my partner he would be better off without me. My close friends have been really supportive but they have their own stuff going on so I keep the full extent of my feeling of despair away from them because I'm sure they are sick of me too. Don't want to go on HRT of AD so I suppose it's my own fault I feel like this.

I've tried herbal stuff, currently trying starflower oil capsules after reading a post about them on this forum. I've upped my exercise regime. I'm vegetarian so try and eat healthily. I've got all the usual aches and pains everyone mentions on this site. I suddenly feel old and I don't like anything about myself anymore. I'm sick of feeling so sorry for myself but I can't seem to get out from under this ever present black cloud. My situation is nothing compared to what some people are going through, and I feel so guilty of feeling so miserable all the time. My palpitations are worse than ever. I've got an ectopic heartbeat so have had all the checks. Can't seem to cope with anything anymore. The slightest thing that goes wrong is like a major trauma now. I never used to be like this.

I'm not sure why I've said all this or what anyone can do. I just feel so alone and thoroughly miserable. I wish someone could wave a magic wand and make things better and make me my previous happy self. I just want all this negativity in my life to stop.

Sorry for whinging. Big hugs to you all x ■

Tiddles
Re: Fed up and so very miserable

Hello Biker Chick. I'm really concerned for you and am sending many virtual hugs across the ether. I was feeling as you are now before taking HRT but only for a few months - a month where I felt life was over during which time I decided to ask for HRT plus the time it took to go through the rigmarole of being prescribed HRT. And then when I started taking it the improvement was rapid (within a couple of days) and remarkable. You mention you can't take HRT because of AD. What is AD? Sorry for my lack of knowledge but I'm newish to the forum and don't understand all the acronyms.

If there's any way you CAN get on HRT you must try it. You can't carry on feeling like this and don't need to xxx ∎

Sammas
Re: Fed up and so very miserable

Hello Biker Chick

Firstly sending hugs. I also know how this feels Hormones take over and nothing is rational I would try something though I am in a dilemma having gone down the natural route, whether to take HRT, as the mood swings, irritability and headaches amongst other things become too much and it's hard to see a light at the end of the tunnel. Everyone is different, but all I would say is you need to try something so you can feel more positive xxx ∎

Dancinggirl
Re: Fed up and so very miserable

Biker Chick - you need a sounding board - so rant away at us if it helps. You sound mentally and physically exhausted so you must see your GP and allow them to help you.
I know exactly how you feel - I came very close to a complete breakdown in my mid 30s - I had started my menopause and my son had just been diagnosed with special needs that would be very challenging. I was lucky as I had a GP at the time that simply took me in hand and told me what I HAD to do. She insisted I have the HRT (thank goodness) and fortunately the practice had a counselor who I saw straight away - I had a year of counseling that has carried me forward really well.
 I am a life vegetarian and was very reluctant to take anything but the GP explained HRT was necessary for my long term health and if you are getting flushes and struggling to sleep I would suggest that a low dose of something like Femoston 1/10 might be worth trying.
You have been through a very traumatic time and your confidence has had a bashing - it's going to take time, practical help and Probably some

medication for you to come out the other side and move forward to enjoy life again.

I had a friend who went through a very bad time and her health was really suffering. Her GP simply told her that her body and mind needed a break, so she agreed to have some ADs for a few months - she took them for just 6 months - and now years later she says it was the best thing she could have done as it allowed her to get her life back on track.

I am not saying you SHOULD take anything but maybe you could consider your options as you simply can't go on like this.

Be kind to yourself. The weather is picking up - get out for some walks in the sunshine - it costs nothing and that vitamin D hit can work wonders.

Keep fighting. DG x ■

Wilks
Re: Fed up and so very miserable

Hi,

Sorry to hear you're feeling so low. I've been there too. I had suicidal feelings for most of last year. I resisted antidepressants for ages but now they (and hrt) have turned me around. I don't know if you can't take them for medical reasons or you just don't want to, but they made me feel like living again.

I also had a great counselor.

If you're not feeling safe, please tell someone or take yourself emergency. ■

paisley
Re: Fed up and so very miserable

Hi

I agree with all that has been said. Depression is a really nasty thing. It robs us of the will to think straight & it is a very lonely place to be in but coming on here & voicing how you feel is good. It gives you a place to vent. I definitely think a trip back to your doctor is in order. That is what they are there for. You might benefit from hrt alone or hrt & AD with some counseling. Talking to someone trained is really good as you can say exactly what you want without being judged. I saw a counselor after I had PND & it really helped. ■

Mary G
Re: Fed up and so very miserable
Biker Chick, I am so sorry to hear about the difficult time you are having. It sounds like you are trapped into a cycle of depression and it is very difficult to break that cycle. My first instinct would be to establish whether or not it is hormonal depression. From what little I know about depression, it seems it can be hormonal, circumstantial (life events) or chemical imbalance and you need to know what you are up against before it can be effectively treated.

My advice would be to go back to your GP as ask for some blood tests, particularly hormones. Then I would consider HRT and/or ADs depending on the results. It could also be worth getting some counseling to help you at this difficult time in your life.

I think the most important thing is for you to find the root cause of your depression and go on from there.

I hope that helps but please do let us know what you decide. ■

Poppi
Re: Fed up and so very miserable

Hi Biker Chick
Big hugs and total understanding, you are not alone in feeling miserable and

sorry for yourself, that doesn't help much immediately but I'm sure tomorrow will be better if you plan to see your GP? I printed off my post for my GP to read and she knew exactly how I was feeling. Now on HRT which suits me. Funny thing, GP was about 30 and just a baby really, but helpful nonetheless. On my way out she recommended I take a look online at the Menopause Matters site as it was fabulous! I never let on!!

Take care   Poppi x ■

Biker Chick
Re: Fed up and so very miserable

Thank you everyone for your supportive comments. I am so glad I found this forum. I am going to go back to my GP, I think I am going to have to give in to either HRT or AD. I have been on the waiting list for therapy with IAPT for 4 months and still haven't heard back from them. I can't go on feeling like this, I'm scared of how bad I am most days. It's ruining my life, my relationship, everything. Thank you to all of you who replied. I am very grateful.

I wish you all well XX ■

Daisydot
Re: Fed up and so very miserable

Hi biker chick you won't regret going on hrt I could have written your post 6 months ago I felt in such a black place and I've had to have some real battles to get where I am now, I still have some issues to resolve but small steps and I know I'll get there, the main thing is I'm 99% improved in every way I just have a few tweaks to make here and there. You go for it life's too short and you have a long journey in front of you still so you may as well try and enjoy living in the day and worry about tomorrow another time. Good luck with gp xx ■

Anonymous
Re: Fed up and so very miserable

Hi

I agree with all that has been said. Depression is a really nasty thing. It robs us of the will to think straight & it is a very lonely place to be in but coming on here & voicing how you feel is good. It gives you a place to vent. I definitely think a trip back to your doctor is in order. That is what they are there for. You might benefit from hrt alone or hrt & AD with some counseling. Talking to someone trained is really good as you can say exactly what you want without being judged. I saw a counselor after I had PND & it really helped ■

English Rose
Re: Fed up and so very miserable

Hello

You sound like you have clinical depression caused by environmental situations and enhanced by hormonal deficiencies.

You must seek help and sometimes that means ADs and HRT. It is not very likely you will come out of the current depression without some sort of intervention be that ADs or hormones. If your body is deficient of any kind of hormone this alone can cause long term health issues with your heart bones and even breast cancers so you owe it to yourself to at least get your hormone levels checked.

I understand not wanting to go on HRT but there are bioidentical HRT (Not synthetics) and these are healthier alternatives to synthetic hormones

Estradiol and Utrogestan (Estrogen and Progesterone) both are bioidentical meaning identical to hormones in our bodies.

The hardest thing to do is reach out and ask for help sometimes.... make the appointment with your doctor take a list of these two hormones and ALL of your symptoms, ask your partner to come with you and remember by helping yourself get better you will also be benefitting those that care about you and live with you as your happiness effects anyone who loves you and lives with you. ■

Biker Chick
Re: Fed up and so very miserable

Hi everyone it's me again. Thank you for today's replies. I will make a note of the names of the bio identical hormones and take them to my GP, thanks for the info English Rose. I suppose waiting 4 months for IAPT is nothing compared to your 33 weeks of waiting Wilks. I'll let you all know how I get on. Thanks again to you all for your support and advice, means a lot xx ■

I think this conversation and the responses are just amazing they serve as a great example of how sharing stories can be so helpful to someone who feels completely alone and out of control! I love all the good advice & support going on here.

PART 8
SYMPTOM CHECKER

There are a lot of charts out there for menopause symptoms, some say there are 34 symptoms, others say 40. The purpose of a chart is to get a clearer understanding of your situation.   Any chart you want to use is great, the one on the next page is included as an example.

SYMPTOM	NONE	SOMETIMES	OFTEN	DAILY
Hot flushes				
Night sweats				
Muscle and joint aches/pains				
Heart palpitations				
Sleep disturbances				
Anxiety				
Difficulty concentrating				
Feeling tense				
Dry or itchy skin				
Vaginal dryness or soreness				
Headaches or migraines				
Brain fog				
Low libido				
Irregular periods				
Thinning hair				
Fatigue				
Bloating				
Fleeing dizzy or faint				
Lethargic and tired				
Unhappy or depressed				
Teary				
Mood changes				
Dry eyes and mouth				
Weight gain				
Frequent & sudden urges to urinate				

PART 10

SOURCES/CREDITS

- https://www.mamamia.com.au/tag/menopause/

- The lesser-known symptoms of menopause no one talks about.

- Article Laura Jackal Contributor - Parenting Dec 5, 2021

- The Secret Power of Menopause By Liza Mundy

- Darcey Steinke - Flash Count Diary: Menopause and the Vindication of Natural Life

- The Slow Moon Climbs: The Science, History, and Meaning of Menopause, by Susan Mattern

- New York Times columnist Gail Collins shows in No Stopping Us Now: The Adventures of Older Women in American History

- https://www.theatlantic.com/magazine/archive/2019/07/work-peak-professional-decline/590650/

- Talking about menopause (finally) - The New York Times Readers react with personal stories of pain and promise, and an ob-gyn shares data. Sept. 22, 2019
- https://www.mommymatters.co/menopause
- https://www.glamour.com/contributor/marisa-mazria-katz
- Early, Unexpected Menopause By Isabel Gillies
- https://www.mysecondspring.ie/stories
- https://www.menopausehub.com
- https://cherokeewomenshealth.com/services/menopause-hormone-therapy/
- https://www.emedicinehealth.com/menopause/article_em.htm
- https://www.wellbeinginfo.org
- https://www.theatlantic.com/author/liza-mundy/
- Facebook Page & Group: Sisters Sharing Stories
- Reddit Group: Sisters Sharing Stories
- https://www.change.org/p/rt-hon-elizabeth-truss-mp-make-menopause-matter-in-healthcare-the-workplace-and-education-makemenopausematter
- https://www.gofundme.com/f/wwwgofundmecomMakeMenopauseMatter
- Davina McCall documentary Sex, Myths And The Menopause
- https://www.irishtimes.com/tags/menopause-society/
- Jennifer Murch - Seven Stories
- https://www.50sense.net/category/menopause-my-story/

- https://www.meno-me.co.nz/real-stories
- https://www.abc.net.au/news/2018-07-16/menopause-the-silent-career-killer/9990252
- https://www.theguardian.com/commentisfree/2020/jan/20/ignorance-menopause-lives-women-information-symptoms
- https://www.evidentlycochrane.com - Everything I needed to know about the menopause… No One Told Me
- https://www.cochrane.org/CD001395/MENSTR_phytoestrogens-for-vasomotor-menopausal-symptoms
- https://www.cochrane.org/CD007244/MENSTR_black-cohosh-cimicifuga-spp.-for-menopausal-symptoms
- Miriam Stoppard's 'Menopause: The Complete Guide to Maintaining Health and Well-being and Managing Your Life'
- https://healthtalk.org/menopause/overview
- https://www.patient.info.com
- https://www.advocacyfocus.org.uk/news/world-menopause-day-our-stories
- https://repeller.com/menopause-symptoms/ article by Jackie Homan
- https://healthandher.com/hot-topics/menopause-and-perimenopause-stories/
- https://www.avogel.co.uk/health/menopause/10-reasons-to-drink-more-water-during-the-menopause/
- https://megsmenopause.com/2020/03/11/a-woman-in-the-mirror/

- https://www.theatlantic.com/magazine/archive/2011/10/the-bitch-is-back/308642/

- *The Wisdom of Menopause*, by Christiane Northrup, M.D.

- https://www.oprah.com/app/o-magazine.html

- https://www.abc.net.au/health/yourstories/stories/2013/06/04/3772930.htm

- https://www.drnancyoreilly.com/is-it-menopause/

- https://time.com/5616247/menopause-expect-messages/

- Suzanne Sommers' - The Sexy Years

- Gail Sheedy's - Silent Passages

- https://hayleysmenopause14.blogspot.com/2020/10/my-story.html

- https://betterafter50.com/category/health/

- https://menopauseunmuted.com/episodes/sharing-stories/transcript

ABOUT THE AUTHOR

Angela Reeves lives in Nova Scotia, Canada. She and her husband Rob recently moved across Canada in pursuit of their long term dream of a farming retirement. They are currently developing their small mixed farm using traditional methods to raise produce, eggs & select livestock, all sold directly off the farm. Not everyone's idea of a relaxing retirement, but they are loving every moment of their busy & active farm life.

This book is Angela's personal passion project and first publication.

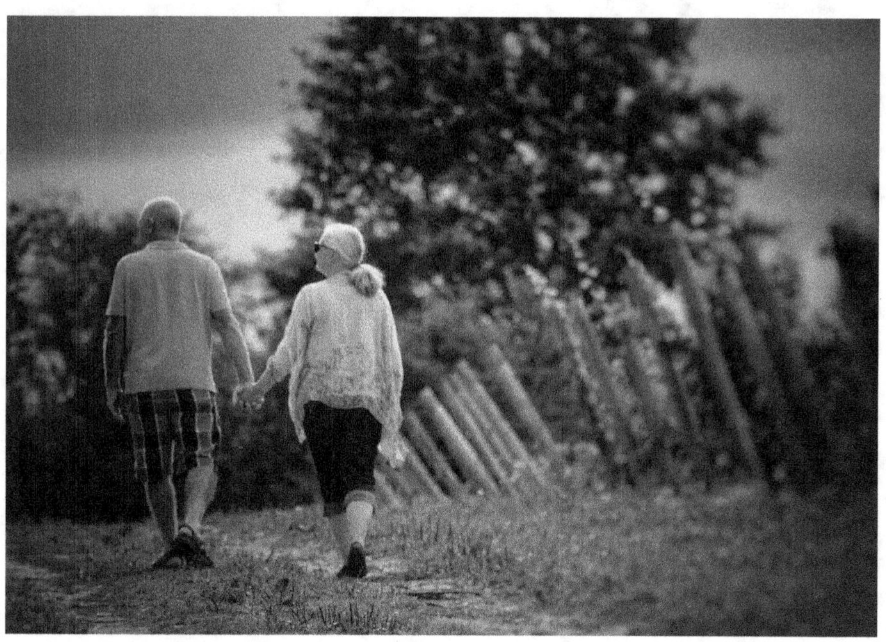

Photo by Kimages find more amazing photos @ www.k-images.ca